**DO NOT REMOVE
CARDS FROM POCKET**

ALLEN COUNTY PUBLIC LIBRARY

FORT WAYNE, INDIANA 46802

You may return this book to any agency, branch,
or bookmobile of the Allen County Public Library.

DEMCO

Caring for the Mentally Impaired Elderly

A Family Guide

Caring for the Mentally Impaired Elderly

A Family Guide

FLORENCE SAFFORD, D.S.W.

HENRY HOLT AND COMPANY • NEW YORK

Copyright © 1986 by Florence Safford
All rights reserved, including the right to reproduce this
book or portions thereof in any form.
First published in January 1987 by
Henry Holt and Company, Inc., 521 Fifth Avenue,
New York, New York 10175.
Distributed in Canada by Fitzhenry & Whiteside Limited,
195 Allstate Parkway, Markham, Ontario L3R 4T8.

Library of Congress Cataloging in Publication Data
Safford, Florence.
Caring for the mentally impaired elderly.
Bibliography: p.
Includes index.
1. Senile dementia—Popular works. 2. Alzheimer's
disease—Popular works. I. Title.
RC524.S24   1986   618.97'689'83   86–11989
ISBN: 0–8050–0080–1

First Edition

Printed in the United States of America
10 9 8 7 6 5 4 3 2 1

ISBN 0-8050-0080-1

This book is dedicated to the memory of my parents, and especially to the memory of my father, whose last years, ravaged by mental deterioration, inspired this book; to my beloved husband, whose wisdom, professional counsel, and constant support made this book possible; and to my daughter, on whom I know I can depend, should I ever become dependent.

CONTENTS

ACKNOWLEDGMENTS

*T*o the many families of the mentally impaired aged who attended my training programs and support groups, my deep appreciation for all that you shared with me.

I am thankful to Lawrence E. Larson, retired executive vice-president of the Isabella Geriatric Center of New York, for the opportunity to develop and implement the first training program for families of the mentally impaired aged.

Above all I would like to acknowledge Rose Dobrof, D.S.W., professor, Hunter College School of Social Work, and executive director of the Brookdale Center on Aging of Hunter College; as mentor, role model, and friend, Rose directed me to the doctoral program of Hunter College School of Social Work, and encouraged the development of my training programs. Her intellectual clarity and breadth, her energy and professional commitment, combine to inspire emulation. I hope that this book proves to be helpful to the elderly and their families, thereby doing justice to her influence.

Caring for the Mentally Impaired Elderly

A Family Guide

Introduction:
My Story

This is not a story with a happy ending, or even a cheerful beginning. It is a chronicle of what can happen to intelligent, competent human beings who are stricken by mental impairment late in life, and what it can do to the families who care for them. But it is much more than a description of deterioration; it is primarily a guide to understanding this very complex problem, and understanding is a first step toward dealing with it.

Alzheimer's disease, or *mental impairment*, is an illness that is often not recognized as such. Commonly known as senility, it can cause embarrassment and shame in a family. Those who have experienced the gradual disintegration of a loved one through the ravages of failing brain cells can attest to the unrelenting pain of this tragedy and to its effect on every aspect of their lives.

How do we begin to describe our feelings at the realization that an aged parent or spouse or brother or sister is showing signs of senility? Can anyone else understand the anguish we feel, the disbelief, the anger, as this capable and independent person steadily changes before our very eyes? Only someone who has had our experience can fully comprehend the pain.

I had spent many years working as a medical social worker and then as a geriatric counselor, helping people solve the problems of their aging relatives, before my own father began to show signs of mental impairment. Only then did I begin to understand the dread of senility and the terrible impact it can have on a family.

My father was a Russian immigrant who came to America at the turn of the century. He struggled throughout his life to gain his independence and then to keep it. Though he had been a musician in Russia, in this country he became a peddler to earn a living. With my mother he managed to open a little store, selling notions and general merchandise in Brooklyn while raising two sons and a daughter. Their business was never successful, but they always told their children that although they were poor, they never turned to charity or welfare. The value of independence was supreme.

Widowed in his late fifties, my father continued alone in his little store, just managing to keep ahead. When he reached the age of sixty-five, he had no plans to retire. In the first place, he was not eligible for social security, since at that time storekeepers were not part of the system, and in the second, he had very little savings. It was a natural assumption that he would keep on working in the store as long as he was able.

By the time he reached his early seventies, my brothers and I became aware that Dad was becoming very forgetful. Often he would have lapses of memory in the middle of telling a story and be unable to continue. We were concerned about his ability to carry on with his store, but we took comfort in knowing that his activities in the store and in his apartment behind the store were so routinized that he could probably perform them without thinking.

A stubborn and irritable man, my father rejected outside help with cleaning and cooking, even though it was very apparent that he required it. So it fell to me, the only daughter, to travel to Brooklyn once a week to clean, shop, and prepare enough food for a week. Between my visits, Dad visited my brothers' homes, and the pattern seemed to satisfy everyone.

When he was in his late seventies, Dad was robbed in his store and beaten when he resisted the robbery. That traumatic event was the turning point in his ability to function independently.

When Dad got out of the hospital, he came to live with me. I was divorced at that time, with a fourteen-year-old daughter. My daughter gave up her room to Grandpa, and we managed for a while in our small apartment without thought of inconvenience or sacrifice.

Although I had been working for some years as director of social services in a large and prestigious home for the aged, I never even considered suggesting to Dad that he become a resident of that home. I was skilled at counseling others and helping them through the difficult decision to place a parent in a home, but I did not recognize that I might have benefited from counseling as well.

Because I wasn't able to face the situation rationally, I made several mistakes. I was unable to assess my father's mental status realistically, and consequently couldn't judge how long he could safely be maintained without supervision. My only concern was whether or not I could deal with his obstinate personality, but since he now seemed defenseless and frail, I felt I could manage. I assumed that my father would stay with me indefinitely, and I proceeded to make moves with long-term consequences.

I bought a house large enough for the three of us and moved in while it was still being renovated. This turned out to be chaotic, since Dad could never remember where to find his room, and the mess of renovation was unbearable, so we moved into a residential hotel while the work was completed. Each move took its toll of my father, whose familiar routines were now gone and who became totally dependent upon me for every activity. By the time we moved into our newly renovated and spacious home, which I selected partly because it was half a block from a senior center, Dad was completely disoriented. Although I was able to drop him off at the senior center before going to work, he sometimes got lost when trying to get home by himself. After being called at work several times to pick him up from the local police station, where he had been taken after wandering for hours in a neighborhood that was utterly strange to him, I knew something would have to be done. Despite my experience, however, I was not able to confront my feelings and formulate any solution. I was so upset that I was not even able to discuss the alternatives with my brothers.

Finally a virtual stranger took control of the situation. The medical director of the geriatric center where I worked, upon learning of my predicament and my father's need for protective care, said authoritatively, "He must come into the home." He then called our affiliated hospital and arranged for a complete medical workup for my father.

By the time Dad was admitted, he was so depleted from the stress of trying to cope in a new environment that he docilely moved into the home, recognizing that help would always be available there. The resistance and anger that I had dreaded never came to pass. His adjustment was immediate. Although he knew no one in the home, everyone looked familiar to him—like so many customers in his little store—and he walked the corridors of his new home safely, greeting everyone as an old acquaintance.

His final five years were spent in comfort at the home. There were many problems, but not for him. In addition to witnessing my father's continuous dissolution, I had to learn to deal with the institutional staff, not just as a colleague but as a responsible relative of one of their charges. I know now that the role of relative to someone in an institution can be one of the most frustrating and challenging of all the roles one plays in a lifetime.

This special perspective led to my intense interest in the dynamics of mental impairment, and my quest for knowledge became the basis of a doctoral project. I developed a training program for other relatives of the mentally impaired aged, both in our institution and in the community at large, so that I could share what I had learned with others who were going through similar turmoil, pain, and guilt.

In the course of seeing my father and running programs for relatives of the mentally impaired aged for several years, I learned more than one ever can from scholarly research alone. This experience is what I would like to share with the readers of this book. I invite you to join me as we set out to examine what is known and unknown about mental impairment in old age, and how you can deal with it in your family.

THE RIDDLE

There is an old riddle that I have shared with many students and members of my training groups for families of the mentally impaired aged: You dream you are in a rowboat with your wife and mother. Suddenly the boat begins to sink, and you realize that you are the only one who can swim, and you can save only one of the two women. What should you do?

Group members and students are always divided in their responses. Some say, "You should save your wife, because she's younger and has a whole life ahead of her. Your mother has already lived a full life, and if she really loved you, she would not want you to sacrifice your spouse for her." Others say, "There's no question but that you should save your mother. You can always get another wife, but you have only one mother." And a few reply, "You had better try to save both, even if you drown in the process, because it would be too hard to go on living anyway if you had let one of them die."

What's the right answer? The answer is: You should wake up. You had *better* wake up, because it is obvious that this is one situation for which there is no solution that will not bring some grief.

In essence, this riddle applies to many people with older loved ones who are mentally impaired. In some cases, what is needed for one member of the family might mean asking excessive sacrifice of others. In other situations, where protective care is imposed on an unwilling older person who is unable to recognize his need, there can be consequences that are just as bad as, or worse than, the original problem. Indeed, it may seem as though all you are doing is trading one set of problems for another.

This book represents my view of what you can do to resolve some of these conflicts.

HOW TO USE THIS BOOK

Reading a book on mental impairment is no substitute for the counseling and advice of professional social workers, nurses, psychologists, and physicians. However, since the extent of this problem has only recently been recognized, you will probably have difficulty in finding professionals who are experienced and educated in the specialization of aging. This book is designed to be used as a guide to help you understand the nature of the problems that face you, and as a personal resource to support you through this ordeal and to reassure you that you are doing the best you can under difficult circumstances. There can be no simple solutions to your problems. Instead, this book provides a perspective that I believe will enable you to sort out your choices more confidently. My goal is to help you develop a level of understanding that will guide you at critical times.

You will notice that I use the male pronoun when I refer to cases and patients. Although there are many more cases where the older patient is female than male (since women live longer), my own personal experience was with a male elderly parent, and so my tendency is to use that pronoun.

You may find some chapters rather technical; but some knowledge of physiology is necessary for a basic understanding of Alzheimer's disease and related mental conditions. The knowledge you gain will help you take a more active role in the care of your relative. But don't worry about remembering all the technical information. It is enough to become familiar with some of the current areas of professional concern.

As you read through the book, you will find some sections more than others applicable to your immediate problems, but as your relative's condition changes, you will find those other sections helpful. By familiarizing yourself with the wide range of issues both in the community and in institutions, you may find directions for the future as well as for your current crisis.

Although you probably feel upset and confused as you start reading this book, I am sure that when you have finished, you will realize that you are not alone with your problems. After considering all of the issues presented, you will be better prepared to make balanced and principled decisions.

1

The Terms of Mental Impairment

When you become aware of mental changes in an older person you love, you can hardly believe it is really happening. At first you look for plausible explanations for obvious memory lapses: "Mother's been worried lately about Dad's health," or "My husband hasn't been himself since his retirement," or "Aunt Rose has been getting more confused and frightened ever since Uncle Joe died." You tend to blame outside forces, because it's too upsetting to face the prospect that your parent or spouse may be falling victim to mental deterioration.

Sometimes it is difficult to describe the changes that

are taking place. You must recognize that something is happening that requires attention, but you may not even know what to call the condition. And not having a name for the alarming process that is taking place certainly can add to your turmoil. In the absence of a more specific diagnosis, let's agree to use the term *mental impairment*.

COMING TO TERMS

What is mental impairment in old age? Is it the same as senility? Is it related to Alzheimer's disease? Is it a mental illness or a psychiatric condition? Don't feel naïve if you have no ready answers to these questions. Even the experts are not in agreement when it comes to naming the condition.

To give you an idea of some of the many names used to describe the condition with which we are concerned, I have assembled the following list of terms from a survey of the professional literature:

> Alzheimer's disease—senile type
> atrophic senile psychosis
> brain damage
> brain dysfunction
> brain failure
> chronic brain syndrome
> cognitive decrement
> cognitive impairment
> confusional state
> delirium
> dementia (degenerative or vascular)
> mental infirmity

mental disorder of the senium
mental impairment
multi-infarct dementia
organic brain syndrome
organic mental syndrome
senile brain disease
senile dementia
senile dementia—Alzheimer's type
senility

You can see for yourself how differently the specialists have viewed the same medical problem.

For the purpose of clarifying the nature of the condition with which we are concerned here, I have chosen to use the term *mental impairment*, because it is the most inclusive as well as the most general, covering the entire range of the disorders listed. Although it may not yet be as widely recognized by the general public as *senility*, which usually refers to mental infirmity in old age and the behavioral changes that accompany it, or *Alzheimer's disease*, the diagnosis that has been garnering so much publicity lately, I feel it is preferable as a neutral term. Its advantage is that it does not have the automatically negative and hopeless connotation of the other terms and it is not so technical that, used diagnostically, it could exclude many causes.

An understanding of the rationale for selecting this term from among the many in use is important, because what we call something often reflects an attitude that can itself have positive or negative effects. Interestingly, even among professionals, there have been swings of opinion as to what to call the condition in old age that causes moderate to severe mental decline, emotional and psychological impairment, and behavioral deterioration. For many years it was called *senile dementia,* and an old person exhibiting symptoms of this mental and behavioral deterioration was said to be demented. As more and more people started living to advanced old age, and as the medical profession began to develop a special interest in geriatrics, the term *dementia* fell into disfavor in the United States, although it continued in use in other parts of the world. American psychiatrists who were working with the aging came to feel that the term was not adequate as a diagnosis for these symptoms.

They noticed that the symptoms fell into recognizable patterns and assumed that these were caused by some physical or organic change in the brain, perhaps a critical loss of brain cells because of the aging process, or damage to brain cells resulting from diminution of the oxygen supply to the brain. The resulting condition came to be called *organic brain syndrome,* a descriptive term indicating that a group of symptoms (a syndrome) was related to physical (organic) changes taking place in the brain.

It was gradually recognized that many of these symptoms were related to specific causes of interference with the availability of oxygen, such as heart failure, infection, anemia, dehydration, malnutrition, and drug toxification, to name just a few. If these conditions were treated, the symptoms could often be reversed. Thus, when organic brain syndrome was identified as being caused by a reversible condition, it was called *acute brain syndrome,* as opposed to *chronic brain syndrome,* which was presumed to be irreversible.

As is customary in medicine, the terms were abbreviated and came to be known as acute or chronic OBS (organic brain syndrome), CBS (chronic brain syndrome), or OMS (organic mental syndrome). Although these terms constitute no more of a diagnosis than does the term *senility*, they were often used as such for the purpose of admitting a confused and disoriented patient to a hospital or to a nursing home.

In time, OBS became an alphabetical label for the behavior, and frequently the labeling resulted in a physician's lack of effort to make a specific diagnosis and lack of interest in considering treatment possibilities. Often doctors attributed the problem of mental decline in the aged to "hardening of the arteries," and advised the family that there was nothing that could be done about it. This was largely because of a negative attitude toward the aging on the part of the medical profession, but it was also due to the time-consuming complexity of determining the cause or causes of the condition.

NEW TECHNOLOGY

In recent years, revolutionary developments in medical technology have led to more enlightened diagnoses. One of these modern miracles is called the CAT (computerized axial tomography) scanner, a new type of X-ray that can show abnormalities in the cells and other parts of the structure of the brain.

Before the CAT scanner, it was possible to examine the condition of the brain only during an autopsy. Today, with this new device, it is possible to examine the brains of the living, and it is now known that similar proportions of brain cells are atrophied or lost during the process of aging by those who are alert as well as by those with impaired mental functions. Clearly, then, it is not just a loss of brain cells that causes the change in mental function; a disease process takes place when mental impairment occurs. With this knowledge, many notions about the effects of aging on the brain have been discarded.

Since the development and availability of the CAT scanner, doctors have been able to determine more easily and precisely those cases in which the mental decline of the older person results from physiological brain damage. This has led to a greater demand for accurate diagnosis, and this concern for diagnosis has, ironically, brought back the use of the term *senile dementia*.

How did this come about? Well, when patients in their forties or fifties developed symptoms of senility, doctors called the condition *pre-senile dementia*, or *Alzheimer's disease*. At the beginning of this century, Dr. Alois Alzheimer studied the brains of young patients who had suffered the same mental and behavioral changes as seen in the aged suffering from senile dementia. He discovered that a large proportion of brain cells seemed to have become atrophied, and he also found some unexpected substances called *plaques*, as well as damage, called *neurofibrillary tangles*, to the nerve cells connecting brain tissue. This condition was named for him, Alzheimer's disease, and since it occurred before age sixty-five, it was also known as pre-senile dementia.

With data now available, it is currently believed that one type of chronic, irreversible dementia that occurs in old age is the same disease as Alzheimer's, with the identical changes in the brain. The only difference is that symptoms develop somewhat later. So the medical community gradually dropped OBS, and the term Alzheimer's disease became the fashion. This condition accounts for over 50 percent of all cases of senile dementia, and is now more often called SDAT (senile dementia of the Alzheimer's type).

OTHER TERMS

With the same new technology, scientists have observed that about 15 percent of cases of senile dementia are caused by the cumulative damage of small strokes, which they are now calling *multi-infarct* (multiple-stroke) *dementia*, or MID. This was previously thought to be cerebral arteriosclerotic disease, or hardening of the arteries of the brain, but evidence from the CAT scanner, as well as new techniques of measuring cerebral blood flow, have led to the conclusion that this type of brain damage is caused by stroke, not by arteriosclerosis. Another 25 percent of the cases are considered the result of a combination of Alzheimer's disease and multi-infarct dementia.

The remaining 10 percent of cases diagnosed as senile dementia are now considered to be acute, temporary symptoms (pseudodementia), which can be reversed if recognized as such and treated promptly.

A WARNING

I still run into professionals who ask, "Whatever happened to OBS?" They are uncomfortable with the generalized use of the term Alzheimer's disease.

And to the layman, arguments over terminology may seem like quibbles. Indeed, at this point you may be asking if this lengthy discussion of terminology has served any useful purpose. Your concern in reading this book is to understand the nature of the problem and to learn how to deal with it. What does it matter what the condition is called? My intent in providing this overview of the fashions in terminology is to offer an insight into the dynamic yet imprecise nature of diagnosing, understanding, and treating this condition. What is important here is to be aware that many doctors today use the terms Alzheimer's disease and dementia just as loosely as others have used the terms senility or OBS. When an elderly person is presented to a doctor with symptoms of mental impairment, all too often the doctor will label it Alzheimer's disease without taking time for the thorough history and testing that are necessary to make an accurate diagnosis.

Of course, this is not true of all doctors. You may have an excellent, caring physician who has properly diagnosed Alzheimer's disease and in whom you can place your trust and confidence. But if you have any reason to doubt the cause of the changes you notice in your relative, you will have to become very observant and learn what questions to ask. And in order to ask questions, you have to know the right words to use.

2

The Symptoms of Mental Impairment

*I*n order to study your relative's behavior for the purpose of helping in the diagnostic process, you have to know what to look for. Even if your relative has already been diagnosed as having an irreversible loss of brain function, you must learn to identify the symptoms of mental impairment in order to learn to cope with them.

You also will want to know as much as possible about what is going on within your relative's brain. You'll want to know what he thinks and feels, and whether he really can't remember or remembers only what he wants to. You'll want to know how aware he is of the problem and how responsible he is for his behavior.

Most of the changes you are seeing in your relative are the results of a disease process that is showing up as a breakdown in the normal functioning of the brain. To recognize these changes, it is important to develop some basic understanding about the brain and how crucial it is in every aspect of our lives.

The brain functions so automatically that we seldom think about it, but in fact it is the physical center of our consciousness, the processor of all our thoughts, and the store of all our memory. It regulates our judgment and our emotions. When the brain begins to fail, the behavior that is affected falls into three categories: *mental changes, emotional changes,* and *behavioral changes.*

MENTAL CHANGES

When we talk about mental changes, we must include all of the processes involved in knowing and awareness: memory, orientation, comprehension, attention and concentration, general information, abstract thinking, judgment and problem-solving skills, and the formation of delusions. Let's look at each one and think about how your relative may be affected by these changes in mental processes.

Memory Loss (Forgetfulness)

As far as memory is concerned, we start out unequally in life; some have excellent memories, others average or below. Some remember names and faces, others music, colors and images, mechanical procedures, spatial relationships, stories, telephone numbers, arithmetic or mathematics, recipes, foreign languages, scientific facts, or current events. Some are brilliant in a few areas and weak in others. Some are average overall.

Whatever the normal level of memory, as we get older, there is usually a gradual failing of memory: names start to elude us; words on the tip of the tongue resist us. It is very embarrassing. Often the names or words come back to us after a while, when we're not consciously trying to remember. This type of memory loss is what we call mild or moderate forgetfulness, or *benign forgetfulness*. This is normal and manageable if we do not panic over it, since anxiety can make it even harder to recall what we are searching for. If we can avoid the nervous reaction to the normal changes in memory that come with age, we can develop ways of compensating, such as written reminders.

Severe forgetfulness, however, is one of the first and most common symptoms of mental impairment in old age. When a person's forgetfulness is serious enough to interfere with his normal functions—for instance, if he cannot remember which food to buy, how to prepare a meal, or even when to eat—he or she can no longer function independently. It is, however, not always a simple matter to determine this and to take appropriate action. The older person whose memory is severely impaired may be too proud to admit it and may cover up with a ready alibi. If you notice that your mother hasn't touched the food you brought earlier in the week, and you question her about it, she might say, "I wasn't hungry, so I didn't prepare anything." This sort of denial is a very common reaction.

Memory can fail in stages. First, the older person may forget people and incidents in an experience. Later, if impairment progresses, the experience itself can be forgotten—leaving a total blank, a kind of amnesia. For instance, the day after attending the celebration of a traditional holiday dinner, an old person may not be able to recall who was there or what was served. As the memory loss becomes more profound, the entire experience of having celebrated the holiday may be forgotten.

Although we will discuss different stages and types of memory loss, you must realize that there are no patterns that are applicable to all older persons who are experiencing these difficulties. This is because there are varying causes of the disorder and each individual responds to these causes in unique ways. There are, however, generally recognizable patterns.

We speak of memory loss in relation to immediate memory, recent memory, and remote or distant memory. Generally, immediate and recent memory are affected first. Forgetting details of an incident that just occurred, not remembering anything from the TV news just seen, not being able to follow an instruction recently given— these are all examples of failure of immediate and recent memory.

As mental impairment gets worse, there may be loss of remote memory, and old remembrances may cease to exist, separating the old person from his past forever. He may forget where he was born, how old he is, or what he did for a living; he may forget his own name or the names of his closest kin. He may not recognize his wife or son, or even himself in a mirror. Previously learned basic skills may be lost, such as simple arithmetic or how to open a can or in what order to put on his clothes. Words are lost, and the ability to express thoughts. Speech may become incomprehensible babble. The medical term for this is *aphasia*.

In later chapters there will be case examples of many of

the problem situations that confront you and your impaired relative and that are attributable to memory loss. At this point it is important simply to recognize serious forgetfulness as a symptom of a disease process.

It is one of the most insidious symptoms affecting all other mental processes, for as the impaired older person loses his memory, he loses his ability to think. He can no longer communicate sensibly. His awareness of himself may disappear, his personality may die.

Be aware, however, that this is *not necessarily the pattern* or terminal state for all problems of memory loss. This is what *may* happen in its most extreme expression. There are some people who can no longer carry on intelligible conversation, but can sing songs. Others can no longer read a newspaper or follow TV, but can still knit beautifully, or build furniture. This variability in how each individual may be affected makes it more difficult for the family to recognize the stages of the illness.

Loss of Orientation

The next significant signs or symptoms of serious mental impairment are those that involve the older person's sense of orientation. The older person may become disoriented about time (what day, hour, or year it is), place (what house or city or country he's in), or person (who you or other people are). In fact, one of the first tests in determining whether someone is mentally impaired is to check his memory by asking such obvious questions as his name and address, his date and place of birth, and what today's date is. The more severe the impairment, the fewer questions the older person can answer.

First to go is the sense of time. A disoriented person

may not only be unaware of what time it is; he may not know if it is early or late, day or night. I remember two residents who used to sit near the entrance of our nursing home, facing a big clock. One day a secretary who was leaving for the day overheard one resident ask the other, "What time is it?" The old lady peered at the big clock, apparently mixed up the big hand and the little hand, and said, "It's twenty-five after eleven. I guess we'll be going to lunch soon." The secretary said, "Excuse me, ladies, but it's five minutes before five o'clock. You'll soon be going to supper." "My goodness," remarked the old lady, "where did the day go?"

Although this lighthearted story shows that some people are not upset by their loss of awareness of time or place, many others do become agitated when they are confronted by this deficit. Indeed, the seriousness of this symptom depends upon its effect on the older person. Some disoriented persons are unaware of their deficit and muddle through the day still able to perform routinized tasks in a restricted and familiar setting, but become disoriented in different surroundings even when these were previously familiar, such as a relative's home. Some older persons are painfully aware of their disorientation and react with fright and anxiety, while others become withdrawn, and still others are able to express their need for reminders, and manage adequately with support from neighbors, friends, and family.

Disorientation is most severe when the older person is not able to remember people. He may recognize someone familiar but not be able to recall the name or the relationship. Eventually he may not even recognize those closest to him.

Another way of describing the symptoms of disorientation is to say that the older person is confused. Confusion results from fragmentation of mental processes, from the inability to make the connections that keep him aware of time, place, or person, from incoherence in thinking; and the word *confusion* is often used by physicians as a diagnosis. But you must remember that confusion is *not* a diagnosis. It is a symptom of memory loss and disorientation, with many possible causes. Those causes must be determined.

Loss of Comprehension

As mental impairment gets worse, the older person may no longer understand what is being said to him, or what he is reading, or even what he is seeing. He may be unable to understand simple instructions, such as, "Wait here. We'll pick you up in ten minutes." This inability to understand an instruction is a stage beyond forgetting it.

The older person may be incapable of understanding how to operate an appliance, or unable to follow instructions regarding his medications. The newspaper may no longer make sense to him; TV programs he used to enjoy may leave him completely confused. New information may not be comprehensible, so he cannot learn, and even things he had previously understood may become incomprehensible.

It is easy to see that the inability to understand can lead to a variety of emotional responses, from passive withdrawal to agitated anxiety. But it may be hard for you to believe that your relative is so impaired, so you may not understand his reactions. If you can recognize your relative's upset behavior as a normal response to a suddenly confusing world, it will become a lot easier to deal with.

Lack of Concentration

As a result of problems with memory and comprehension, there is usually a change in the older person's ability to concentrate; lack of attention is a frequent early sign of mental impairment. There is a noticeable reduction in the person's attention span. The older person may be easily distracted and unable to muster enough attention to take part in normal conversation or discussion, or follow a train of thought. This can lead to stereotyped repetition of a few ideas, over and over again, without regard to their relevance in conversation.

It sometimes happens that an older person is able to understand or comprehend but has lost the ability to concentrate sufficiently to be able to absorb and integrate what is going on about him. If you have noticed this with your relative, it is important to observe whether his difficulty with concentration varies with his energy level or is more pronounced at one time of day than another. This information could be of use in structuring a more supportive environment for the older person, as we will see in a later chapter.

Loss of General Information

One of the symptoms of mental impairment that is not always as noticeable as the others is the loss of general information. It may not be apparent in ordinary, day-to-day interaction, but the older person may no longer know who is the mayor of his city or the president of the country. The first kind of general information that typically eludes him is of recent origin, such as current events, but as mental impairment progresses, old and commonly known facts will disappear as well. An example of this latter loss would be the inability to remember what holiday is associated with Santa Claus or matzoh or jelly beans.

If the older person is aware of this loss of general information, he may try to conceal it by humorous quips, somehow maintaining that he is still aware of his environment. I recall one old person who was asked if she knew who was currently President of the United States. She replied with a twinkle in her eye, "I don't remember his name, and I don't even know what he looks like. But I know he's a regular humpty-dumpty, just like all other politicians."

An alternative reaction might be a withdrawal from painful, embarrassing contacts. Still another common reaction to the sudden awareness of no longer knowing basic facts of everyday life is an agitated state of anxiety, with the terrified old person declaring, "I must be losing my mind."

Loss of Insight and Logic

In some cases, even though the older person is still able to understand what is being said to him, he may lose the ability to think abstractly. With advancing impairment, the mental connections needed to think abstractly may break down, making it impossible for the older person to take part in anything but the simplest, most concrete conversation. For example, you may say to your relative, "It's a lovely day today. Let's go for a walk," but he may not understand the connection between a lovely day and taking a walk. It might be easier for him if you said simply, "Let's go for a walk."

With only concrete thoughts available, the older person is no longer capable of insight, which is an internal way of understanding a situation or of understanding oneself in relation to others. The person who lacks insight may be preoccupied with himself and unaware of the needs and feelings of those close to him.

The mental process of logic is dependent on the ability to make connections between ideas or facts, to make inferences that lead to rational thinking and reasonable behavior. You can see that logic is lost to the older person who is no longer able to think abstractly. Furthermore, the older person who is limited to concrete thoughts is unable to put together the information needed for day-to-day problem solving.

Loss of Judgment

Related to the loss of insight is the loss of judgment. You may not recognize faulty judgment as a symptom of mental impairment, although it can be a very serious impediment to an older person's ability to care for himself. The loss of this significant mental process interferes with the older person's normal ability to make the ordinary decisions necessary for safety and good health and to use the problem-solving skills accumulated during the experience of a lifetime. For example, the older person who goes outdoors in very cold weather wearing inappropriate clothing demonstrates that he no longer has the judgment to decide what to wear in relation to the climate. People can make mistakes in judgment all through their lives, but when poor judgment reflects errors based upon normally simple associations, it is then a symptom of an illness. This mental loss affects such potentially hazardous areas as the ability to drive a car, to handle finances, or to protect oneself from crime.

It is a particularly difficult problem for families when this loss of judgment makes it impossible for the older person to recognize and accept the need for protective care.

Formation of Delusions

In some impaired older persons, the disordered thoughts that result from loss of memory, confusion, disorientation, lack of judgment, and other distorted mental processes lead to the formation of delusions. With loss of insight and of the ability to distinguish between real events and thoughts, delusions may occur. The older person who experiences delusions believes them to be true, even though they may be bizarre and blatantly impossible. These may be visual delusions, in which the older person sees something no one else sees (a cat in the room) or auditory delusions, in which the older person hears something no one else hears (voices telling him something). Or the older person may develop a system of ideas that explains events which otherwise have not made sense to him (such as that Martians have landed on Earth).

All of these examples will be discussed fully in later chapters as the day-to-day problems are examined in detail.

EMOTIONAL CHANGES

It is obvious that people who are even partially aware of their mental losses will respond with many emotions, such as fear, anger, frustration, sadness, hostility, and depression. These emotional reactions may appear in addition to similar symptoms caused by organic brain changes.

There can be many emotional and personality changes taking place that are directly caused by impaired brain function and must be recognized as symptoms of this disorder, but they are often interpreted as normal for the aged, and are therefore resented and criticized. Throughout the examples I will present of problem situations, I will be reminding you to recognize the changes as symptoms of a disorder, not as difficult personality traits. Sometimes these changes are *responses* to the mental changes taking place and sometimes they are the direct result of changes in brain function.

Emotional behavior is complex; it involves physiological, biological, and chemical responses to outside events and interpersonal situations. These responses are processed by particular centers in the brain. Impaired functioning of any part of the chain of reactions can trigger an unusual emotional response.

Some of the most common personality changes you may notice are the following:

Emotional Lability

This is the psychological term that describes the loss of emotional control, and it frequently accompanies the mental losses of the impaired older person. The emotionally labile person will be subject to fits of crying or laughing, usually inappropriately. You may notice mood swings. There may be sudden outbursts of temper or rage out of proportion to the event that caused them. When this represents a change from the older person's normal behavior, it should be viewed as a symptom of some organic or physical change taking place and reported to a physician.

If this happens to your relative, you may find yourself

reacting emotionally, too. It's not easy in the midst of an emotional scene to remind yourself that it's a symptom, and not to overreact. But you will learn, as you study this book, to train yourself to remember that it is a symptom of mental changes your relative can't control.

Lack of Emotional Response

Sometimes the change is the opposite of emotional lability. The psychological term used to describe an inappropriate decrease in emotion is *flatness of affect*. Your relative may seem apathetic, unable to respond with normal animation. He may appear withdrawn. He may be incapable of feeling happy when something pleasant has occurred, and incapable of expressing sadness or anger when these emotions would be normal. There might seem to be a dullness of mood, which can be interpreted as depression, but if you ask if he is upset or unhappy, he will probably respond that he is not. This can be as difficult a symptom to deal with as the outbursts of the labile person, since your relative may be unresponsive to all efforts to please him.

Anxiety

If your relative is aware of some mental changes taking place in him, he may become frightened and develop anxiety about it. The anxiety itself can make the symptoms worse. Anxiety can be a perfectly normal response to signs of illness, and it is sometimes relieved by understanding and reassurance.

It can also be caused by some breakdown in the function of the brain and central nervous system. It can lead to many behavioral changes that are difficult to deal with, such as irritability or nervousness and agitation. Anxiety can prevent the older person from carrying out the normal day-to-day activities he would otherwise still be capable of handling. However, it is a symptom that may be relieved by the right medication. This will be discussed in chapter 9.

Irritability

This is another emotional behavior that has many possible causes. Irritability is a way of expressing a generalized feeling of anger, which can be directed at anything or anyone available. It can be viewed as a symptom of mental impairment when it is out of proportion to the situation that provokes it and when it represents a change in the older person's usual way of behaving. It may also be a symptom if there are other signs of mental impairment, such as memory loss, confusion, and disorientation. Irritability is an ironic symptom. It reflects a state of emotional discomfort that cries out for help, but often it alienates those who would like to help. It should be easier for you to accept your relative's irritability when you recognize it as a sign of impaired brain cell function, a symptom he cannot control.

Hostility

When the anger experienced by the impaired person is projected toward those around him, it is sometimes expressed as open hostility. This hostility may take the form of snide remarks, verbal attacks, belligerence, or even physical aggression.

Many family members feel very hurt and offended

when they are insulted by their impaired relatives. It is most important for those care-givers who are the target of hostility to remember that their relative is responding emotionally to situations he is no longer able to understand.

All of us have hostile impulses when we feel frustrated or threatened. As part of growing up, we are taught to repress those impulses. Unfortunately, if the part of the brain that has learned to control such impulses becomes impaired, instinctive hostility can come through when an older person feels personally attacked or overwhelmed. The hostile response is your relative's primitive way of trying to protect himself. As the relative of a hostile, belligerent, or aggressive older person, you must be on guard to avoid responding with anger. This is extremely difficult, but it is a challenge you must try to meet.

Stubbornness

Another difficult change in personality that may appear as a symptom of mental impairment is stubbornness. It is often a characteristic of those who are trying to maintain their sense of control over their own lives as their capacity for independence is slipping away. With the loss of insight, the older person may be unaware of the inappropriateness of his stubborn behavior in relation to those who are trying to be helpful.

Stubborn, obstinate behavior, which can take many forms, often shows up as an insistence on "being right." This is often a very frustrating area for family members. Many of you will nod in agreement when I tell you how upsetting it is when your relative stubbornly refuses a bath, saying he had one already. No amount of logical reasoning will get through to him. Or your relative may insist on going someplace when it is not appropriate or safe, and he will stubbornly demand that he be allowed to do as he wants. If the stubborn impaired person feels too frustrated, he might have a temper tantrum or do something destructive.

Many members of the family groups I've met have described their feelings of helplessness when they found themselves arguing with relatives who insisted that they were "right" in spite of the facts. They felt that they were stooping to the level of their relative by trying to prove he was "wrong," but they were not always able to stop. If it can be seen that the stubborn behavior stems from the older person's need for self-esteem and his dual loss of awareness of the roles of others and of insight, then it becomes easier to deal with the behavior. Try to avoid arguing with someone whose stubbornness is beyond reasoning.

Loss of Sense of Humor

Many older persons are able to maintain a good façade, despite serious mental impairment, through a habitual pattern of humor. They may rationalize their loss of memory with humorous quips, poking fun at themselves or at others. They may use their sense of humor as a means of quelling some of their anxiety.

Others may experience a total personality change and lose their customary sense of humor, and this represents another level of loss of brain function. Here the older person is no longer able to understand as humorous something that someone else has said, or may lose the skill of handling social interactions lightly and with fun. The ability to find humor in situations requires a level of abstraction that may no longer be available in the older person's repertoire of mental skills.

Suspiciousness

When the older person is no longer in control of his environment and cannot understand the changes that are taking place, he may blame others for the changes. He may suspect that someone close to him, or even a stranger, is responsible for his difficulties. Thus, if he misplaces items and cannot remember handling them, he may think that someone else misplaced them.

Some of you may have a relative who hides things for safekeeping and later cannot remember where he hid them, or even that he hid them in the first place. Very often, such a person becomes convinced someone else must have lost or stolen the items because he has absolutely no recollection of having put them away.

Sometimes the suspicious reaction to unexplainable events may seem to be a continuation or exaggeration of a previous personality trait. It would be the degree of suspiciousness in relation to the actual occurrence that would indicate if it might be a symptom of changes of brain function. At other times the trait of suspiciousness may appear unexpectedly, in a previously trusting relationship. Then it is easier to detect as a symptom.

Jealousy

At times the suspicious older person may experience irrational jealousy. You may be startled one day to find that your relative is sullen, insulted by something you have failed to do. I remember one relative whose mother accused her of working just so that she wouldn't have to spend so much time with her. In fact, the daughter was a lawyer and she had been working full time all her adult life. The impaired mother no longer remembered that her daughter was a busy professional. She could only express jealous anger that the daughter was not with her as much as she wanted.

Sometimes the previously independent older person will complain petulantly, or possibly fly into a jealous rage, when he feels that you are favoring someone else in the family over him. This behavior can even take the unreasonable form of complaining that you pay more attention to your child or spouse than to your older relative.

Jealous behavior is also a symptom, reflecting a loss of judgment or insight, or of the ability to understand the behavior of others. It may also reflect damage to the part of the brain that controls our emotional reactions. Many of us experience jealous reactions in everyday situations, but as part of growing up we have learned to control these. Social maturity involves the storing of acceptable responses in the brain that cancel out primitive jealous responses, which we learn are "not nice." Although the feelings may be experienced throughout our lives, they are kept in check (for the most part) by automatic learned controls. If the brain center that controls this learned response becomes impaired, the older person may exhibit childish jealous reactions to normal situations. These can be very upsetting to those around him unless they are recognized as a symptom of pathology of the brain.

Paranoia

When the suspicious older person becomes convinced that others are responsible for the problem he is having, despite any verifiable evidence, we may say that this extreme reaction is a symptom of *paranoia*. Paranoia is partly the result of anxiety over what is no longer understandable for the impaired person, and it causes alarm to relatives who must respond to the distorted ideas. This disturbed, disordered thinking process presents some of the most difficult problems for the family of the older person, as well as to professional care-givers.

Paranoia can be considered a symptom of general mental impairment, or it can be a distinct mental illness, related to organic or chemical changes in a specific part of the brain. It can appear with or without other severe mental changes. It is often related to sensory losses, such as those of hearing or vision, and may be seen as the older person's attempt to understand the distortions he now perceives as his normal environment.

Whatever the reason for the paranoid thinking, it baffles and upsets family members who must deal with it. Is there anything more painful than to be accused of stealing from someone whose well-being means so much to you?

Paranoia is such a significant problem area that I have devoted an entire chapter (chapter 7) to it.

BEHAVIORAL CHANGES

Just as it is important for you to recognize certain emotional and personality changes as symptoms of impaired brain function, so must you learn which changes in behavior may be symptomatic of mental impairment. It is much more difficult to see a cause-and-effect relationship between brain failure and behavioral problems, but I am sure you will readily see a relationship between some of the mental and emotional symptoms already described and the behavioral characteristics that follow.

Some of the most common changes you may see in your relative's behavior are the following:

Loss of Initiative

A frequent sign of advancing mental impairment is a loss of initiative or ability to start actions independently. For example, your mother may ask, all day long, "What should I do now?" This is a call for help from a previously independent person who was accustomed to being busy and now needs direction for most activities. You may first notice this change as a lack of spontaneity, as the impaired person seems to lose the capacity to make plans. You may feel that your relative has become immobilized, bound to the immediate situation, unable to think through what he should do.

Inability to Follow Through

Many of you may have relatives who are able to initiate activities but get stuck in the middle and can't finish. When the brain falters in making the automatic connections from one thought to the next, the older person is unable to complete a meaningful action. He becomes confused about what he is doing and why.

This is the extreme form of the early memory problem. At the stage where memory failure is benign, the individual retraces his steps mentally to reconstruct what he was doing and, through logic, remembers what he wanted to do. The mentally impaired older person no longer has the ability to reconstruct a mental process. He cannot make the connection from one thought to the next. It is too complex a task. His mind draws a blank. This is the basis for many changes in behavior.

Loss of Interest

When an impaired older person is no longer able to initiate his own activities, or becomes unable to follow through his activities to completion, he often withdraws from social relationships. He seems to lose interest in what's going on. He may not even seem to pay attention to family matters or to anything that had once been of interest. He may seem unresponsive or apathetic.

This behavior may be viewed as a normal reaction to an abnormal condition—that is, to the state of being mentally impaired. It can be a way of adapting to the inability of the brain to handle its usual tasks. Or it may result directly from impaired thinking, as the brain is incapable of making the connections between concepts.

It is very important to consider whether your relative's apathetic behavior may be a sign of depression rather than of mental deterioration, or whether he is depressed in addition to the other symptoms of impairment. You can help in the diagnostic process by observing your relative's moods and reporting whether he seems sad or not. Your observations can result in different treatment for your relative.

Personal Neglect

Sometimes the first clues you may have to the serious extent of mental changes that have taken place are signs of neglect in your previously well-groomed relative. If your relative is inattentive to his environment, he may also fail to notice his soiled tie or dirty sweater. If he is unable to initiate or complete a task, he may be unable to take a bath or to dress himself properly. Combing his hair or brushing his teeth may prove to be too much of a challenge to his failing mind.

The older person who is made aware of these areas of neglect is usually embarrassed, and often he denies the obvious. This may prove to be one of the really challenging problems for you, calling for sensitivity and tact, and imagination in finding practical solutions. For more about personal hygiene, see chapter 8.

Restlessness

In contrast to the withdrawn, apathetic behavior we have already discussed, some confused, forgetful older people may become restless or hyperactive. It is very common to find impaired older people who constantly rummage through drawers or closets looking for something but not having any idea what they are looking for. You may find your relative shuffling papers on a desk, apparently sorting and organizing but in reality simply moving them around. Others may push around pieces of furniture or pick up objects from tables or shelves and place them elsewhere. This incessant shuffling and rummaging can lead to the misplacement of many items and the unintentional confiscation of others' belongings.

The need to be active and the inability to follow through a purposeful activity can lead to wandering behavior. The older person moves around aimlessly, not knowing where he wants to go or how to get there, at home or elsewhere, and is in constant danger of wandering out into a corridor or street or other area that is strange to him. This will be discussed further in chapter 6.

Verbal Changes

You may find that although your relative seems to be alert, it is difficult for you to understand what he is trying to tell you. He may start out saying something relevant, but as he continues, unrelated phrases seem to creep in. This is what happens when some older persons, somewhat aware of their gaps in memory, attempt to correct this by inventing stories. These are usually a mixture of fantasy and incidents in their remote memory. Although you may find this irritating, you must realize that it is not done consciously, for the older person usually cannot distinguish the fantasy from reality. This is called *confabulation* and can be understood as the confused older person's attempt to compensate for the blank parts of his memory.

Another verbal pattern that may appear is called *perseveration*, in which the impaired person may become repetitious in response to the few thoughts now available to him, and constantly state the same facts. I remember one resident in our geriatric center who always greeted everyone by saying, "In my day we weren't afraid of hard work. I worked sixteen hours a day, seven days a week. If you have anything to do, don't be afraid to call on me."

As the older person's concentration fails and he is not able to hold his thoughts together to complete a meaningful statement, he may ramble on. He may start to answer a question appropriately but then get carried away by his thought processes, forgetting the original question, and talk on and on.

Still another behavior that may appear is *irrelevant con-*

versation, in which the older person who seems to be socially involved may respond to a situation with a statement that has nothing to do with what has been said before. This may happen because the older person is used to taking part in social conversation, but no longer has the ability to understand the nature of the conversation. Or it may be that he understands the conversation but no longer can put the words and thoughts together to respond coherently.

Some family members are intuitively able to understand what their relatives are trying to say, and can help them express it. Others need to develop skills in interpreting their relative's new language.

Loosening of Inhibitions

The maintenance of good manners and appropriate behavior requires an awareness of what is expected in the presence of others. When function fails in the centers of the brain that control learned social behavior, the mentally impaired older person may display uninhibited behavior, which can be embarrassing and upsetting to others. For example, when he feels the urge to go to the bathroom, your relative may start to open his pants wherever he is, uninhibited by the presence of others.

Or an old person who was normally polite and tactful may make insensitive comments to others.

I remember a member of one of my groups who told of wanting to die of embarrassment every time she had guests, even when they were other relatives. Her husband would always say tactless things like, "Why do you come here? You're too ugly," or "Fat people are slobs. Go away. I don't like you." The loss of inhibition also may account for aggressive behavior in a previously polite, mild-mannered person.

Sometimes family members are shocked by the abusive and vulgar language that can be used by someone who has been a model of dignity and proper behavior. Even when the behavior is recognized as a symptom of mental impairment, you will find it difficult to understand if it happens to your relative.

The aspect of loss of inhibitions that is most difficult to cope with involves sexual impulses. The impaired older person may start to handle his genitalia or masturbate publicly or make inappropriate sexual advances to others. This behavior must also be understood as a symptom of mental impairment, and will be discussed in chapter 8.

Impulsiveness

When someone who has usually behaved in a mature and rational manner beings to behave impulsively, it may also be a symptom of mental change. The change may not be noticeable unless it is related to imprudent decisions. The older person may buy things he can't afford or make excessive gifts or donations. Or he may become involved in social relationships that cause his family concern. If this is happening to your relative, you must learn that sometimes this behavior is a cue that he is in need of some kind of protective care. This will be discussed in chapters 6, 7, and 10.

Hoarding

In some cases, a distorted mental state will express itself in hoarding behavior. The older person seems to develop a compulsion to accumulate and save things, often things without any apparent value. Newspapers and magazines may be collected until they become a safety hazard in a household. Food may be stored in the refrigerator even after it turns moldy or rancid. Junk may be collected from other people's discarded garbage.

Some experiments with animals have shown that stimulation of a specific part of the brain (the hypothalamus) may cause hoarding behavior. While it is not known what causes this behavior in humans, it is possible that it is related to damage to a specific area of the brain in the mentally impaired aged. The hoarding behavior seems to serve some emotional need, probably an anxious reaction to their confusion. Understanding the basis of the behavior is important in learning how to cope with the problems it may create.

For example, if you recognize that some emotional anxiety is causing your relative to hoard things, you should try to let him know that you can understand his feelings and that you want to help him. Instead of criticizing him for collecting junk or causing a hazardous condition, by recognizing his feelings you may be able to get his cooperation in discarding some of the collection.

Perceptual Changes

Among the many possible changes in behavior you may observe in a mentally impaired older person are those related to faulty perceptions of what he sees, hears, feels, or senses. Since all of our sensory experiences depend upon appropriate brain activity, it should be apparent that if there is impairment in the part of the brain that receives impulses from the senses, then those impulses will not be registered correctly and acted upon.

The word *perception* describes the very complex process of how we organize, integrate, and respond to stimuli we receive through our senses. Correct perceptions require: (1) healthy eyes, ears, taste buds, sense of smell, touch receptors, sense of warmth or cold, and sense of balance; (2) a healthy nervous sytem to transmit these sensations to the appropriate part of the brain; and (3) healthy brain activity.

Many older persons experience a physical decline as they age, with failing eyesight, hearing, taste sensation, and so on. If your relative is showing signs of changes in any of these sensory areas, and if there is no apparent physical reason, then it is very likely related to impaired mental function.

Incontinence

When someone loses bladder or bowel control, he is said to be incontinent of urine or feces. The problem of incontinence may be related to purely physical changes, or it may be due to loss of brain function. Since this area is highly charged emotionally, causing embarrassment for all involved, it is sometimes very difficult to determine the source of the problem. It is essential to assist your relative in obtaining a thorough examination, since his embarrassment and/or mental impairment may interfere with his ability to cooperate sufficiently for a physician to make an accurate diagnosis. If there is no physiological reason for the incontinence—such as prostate enlargement or urinary tract infection—it would probably be related to mental impairment.

This is one of the most difficult problems for families to deal with, and often is the basis for a decision to place the older person in a nursing home. Incontinence is discussed at length in chapter 8.

Up to this point I have tried to explain the nature of mental impairment in old age as a disease process, by describing many of the symptoms it may present. The next chapter will discuss the many possible causes of this complex condition.

3

The Causes of Mental Impairment

*A*lthough many promising advances have been made in recent years in studies of the structure and activity of the brain, it is still not known specifically what causes its functions to break down. Mental impairment is related to the destruction of brain cells and a failure in the mechanics of transmitting messages from one cell to another, but we still do not know what destroys the cells or disrupts the transmission of messages. We are dealing with the phenomenon of brain damage, or brain failure, with many possible causes and effects.

In chapter 1, I explained that conditions that cause

mental impairment are either *acute* and possibly reversible with treatment, or *chronic*, with no known cure. The causes of reversible mental impairment are no more easily identifiable, and will be discussed in the latter section of this chapter. But first let's review what is known about the disease believed to be the most common cause of chronic mental impairment.

SENILE DEMENTIA—ALZHEIMER'S TYPE

Alzheimer's disease presents characteristic changes in the structure of the brain as well as in its metabolism or biochemistry, and in the amount of blood flowing to it. Some changes can be seen with the CAT scanner, while others can be seen only under a microscope.

Brain Structure

The brain damage seen in victims of Alzheimer's disease is a destruction of brain cells that leaves scars, which have been described as *plaques* and *tangles*. The plaques are a waxy substance; they may be the result of an abnormal breakdown of proteins deposited in the nerve cell. In other cells, there is some kind of granular degeneration in the center. The tangles, known technically as *neurofibrillary tangles*, appear to be twisted filaments of nerve cell endings. Scientists believe that they are the result of physical or chemical damage to the brain. For example, when prize-fighters sustain serious or repeated injuries to the head, they sometimes develop symptoms of slowness in thinking and speech and unsteadiness in walking (they're called "punch drunk"). On examination, their brains show the same "tangles" that are found in Alzheimer's disease. It's assumed that when they are injured, physical trauma either damages the brain directly or starts a chain of chemical changes that results in the same "tangles" characteristic of Alzheimer's disease. We do not know what actually causes the damage, however.

Brain Metabolism or Biochemistry

For the brain to function normally, it must have a constant flow of healthy blood to supply oxygen, glucose, and other nutrients. Certain enzymes or chemicals called *neurotransmitters* carry impulses or messages from one cell to another. One of the most common neurotransmitters is *acetylcholine*, found in the part of the brain that controls intellect and emotion. The action of the neurotransmitter is speeded up by an enzyme secreted by specific nerve cells, which acts as a catalyst. For acetylcholine to be metabolized effectively in transmitting messages, the enzyme *choline acetyl transferase* is produced by the appropriate neurons in the brain.

Through the amazing techniques that have recently been invented, it has been found that there is a marked decrease of choline acetyl transferase activity in the brains of people with Alzheimer's disease. The more severe the symptoms of Alzheimer's disease, the greater the loss of that enzyme activity. It has also been found that this does *not* occur in cases of other types of senile dementia, such as multi-infarct dementia, where a different type of brain damage is seen.

In addition, it is known that the metabolization of acetylcholine is dependent upon the amount of oxygen available. This is an important point to keep in mind, considering the early idea that lack of oxygen to the brain was one of the major causes of the condition that was called "organic brain syndrome."

Cerebral Blood Flow

With the new techniques developed to measure the flow of blood in the brain, which also make it possible to track the direction it goes during specific mental functions, doctors can now see how much of the brain is functioning and locate the changes in function.

For example, when a healthy person is asked to do some calculations, there is an increase in the amount of blood flow to the right side of the brain. The more severe the degree of intellectual impairment, the less blood flows to the brain. Doctors have found that the overall amount of blood flow to the brain is decreased in senile dementia, and the ability to initiate or activate an increased supply when a specific task demands it is also decreased.

How does all of this technical information help us in understanding Alzheimer's disease?

It should be easy to see that there is a relationship between the structural changes (the plaques and tangles), the metabolic changes (speed of transmission of impulses between neurons), and the change in cerebral blood flow if we realize that how we think and behave is dependent upon (1) the number of healthy brain cells available; (2) the amount of oxygen and glucose supplied to specific parts of the brain; and (3) the speed with which messages are transmitted from one brain cell to another. Just how they are related in terms of cause and effect still eludes the scientific community, but it is getting closer to the answers every day. It is, for example, possible that the plaques and tangles interfere with the transmission of neural impulses by slowing them down or blocking them altogether. It is also possible that the plaques and tangles interfere with the process through which nutrients are delivered to the nerve cells, which would in turn disrupt thought processes.

Locating the Damage

It appears that these pathological changes occur first in the part of the brain that is responsible for short-term memory (the hippocampus). In later stages of the disease, these changes involve the parts of the brain responsible for emotional and intellectual function (the limbic area and the entire cerebral cortex). Keep this in mind and you will recognize that as the damage to the brain increases and spreads to larger and different areas, you will see increasing symptoms of forgetfulness, and then total mental deterioration and emotional changes.

Most people know that the brain depends constantly on oxygen and that with a decrease in the flow of blood to the brain there will be a decrease in the supply of oxygen. You should also know that the synthesis of the neurotransmitter acetylcholine is negatively affected by a lack of oxygen. Therefore, the changes that scientists have found in the neurotransmitters may be the result of a decrease in oxygen. Or it may be that the decrease in oxygen is the result of slowing down or inactivity of the neurotransmitters, which therefore would demand less blood. As yet, the nature of the relationship is not known.

There remains the nagging question of what causes the breakdown of nerve cells that secrete choline acetyl transferase, and what causes the cell damage that results in plaques and tangles. If it is related to decreased oxygen supply or lack of glucose or other nutrients, why does it occur only in specific areas of the brain?

Some Current Theories

It appears that part of the answer lies in our genes. Scientists believe that we inherit a predisposition to particular characteristics, both physical and psychological. Our genes dictate a pattern for our development and decline, but they are influenced by environmental and social factors. What we eat and drink, how it is absorbed and eliminated, what drugs we take, how much we exercise, what we feel about ourselves—all have a profound impact on how our genetic program is fulfilled. However, if we accept the concept of a biological clock that is timed for specific physical changes regardless of external influence, then we must accept the fact that certain physiological breakdowns, including brain failure, will occur if our genes so dictate.

Among the other theories about the causes of Alzheimer's disease, scientists are working on the possibility that it is the result of some latent, slow-acting virus that may be in the system for years, finally causing the breakdown in function of brain cells. They are also studying the effects of toxins in the system; for instance, high concentrations of aluminum have been found in the brains of Alzheimer's disease victims. Here again the issue of cause and effect is basic to the investigation, as scientists do not know whether excess aluminum might cause cell damage, or whether it is the residue after brain cell damage has occurred.

One last significant area of investigation is based on

the theory that the type of brain cell damage characteristic of Alzheimer's disease may result from a breakdown of the body's immune system. It is thought that through some genetic error the immune system may destroy the body's own healthy cells, damaging the cells' ability to manufacture enzymes and proteins.

These theories are all tentative and exploratory, each attacking this complex disease from a different angle, yet all may be related in some way. We must accept the fact that although an amazing amount of new knowledge about the possible causes of Alzheimer's disease is beginning to accumulate, there is still much that we do not know.

MULTI-INFARCT DEMENTIA

There is a category of mental impairment that is now believed to be the result of accumulated damage to the brain caused by multiple strokes over a period of time.

What is a stroke? When the blood supply to the brain is cut off by a spasm, the rupture of an artery, a blockage, or arteriosclerosis (hardening of the arteries), a stroke occurs. A stroke, also called a *cerebral vascular accident* (CVA), can be the result of an embolism (a traveling blood clot), a thrombosis (a clot formed locally in an artery), or an aneurysm (rupture of a weak blood vessel). The resulting damage to brain tissue that has been deprived of oxygen is called a *cerebral infarct* or *infarction*.

The appearance of such tissue when it occurs in the brain has been described as "cerebral softening," and it can be seen through the CAT scanner. This disease process is now called *multi-infarct dementia*, which identifies its source as brain damage from multiple strokes, and is sometimes called *arteriosclerotic dementia*.

It was previously believed to be the result of cerebral hardening of the arteries, but new techniques have led to the current belief that it is related to atherosclerosis (narrowing of the arteries) in other parts of the body, although there is also greater incidence of cerebral arteriosclerosis than is found in victims of Alzheimer's disease.

Symptoms

Multi-infarct dementia can be diagnosed by physicians from studies of the brain as well as from a history of the mental and physical changes that have occurred. Whereas the mental impairment resulting from Alzheimer's disease is a slowly appearing condition that gets steadily and progressively worse over a period of years, the mental impairment that results from multi-infarct dementia usually appears suddenly and proceeds irregularly. The severity of the symptoms is related to the accumulation of damage from the strokes as they occur. Since new areas of the brain can sometimes pick up the function of the damaged areas, the symptoms may clear up. Improvement may be possible, and then new damage may develop, resulting in what doctors describe as a *stepwise course* of the disease.

As in Alzheimer's disease, the symptoms of multi-infarct dementia are related to the areas of the brain in which cell damage appears. However, while damage in Alzheimer's disease seems to occur symmetrically in both the right and left sides of the brain, multi-infarct damage usually appears only on one side of the brain, which can be identified by the physician from the mental and physical symptoms.

This difference in diagnosis is most important in possible treatment, since future strokes might be prevented and further deterioration avoided. Good medical care in preventing strokes would include: (1) means to reduce high blood pressure, (2) treatment of heart conditions, (3) treatment of peripheral vascular disease, and (4) attention to diabetes. This preventive regimen might include diet and exercise, medication, and possibly even vascular surgery to improve circulation.

Little Strokes

It is important for the family to watch for evidence of "little strokes," or transient ischemic attacks (TIAs). These can range from barely noticeable occurrences—mild, temporary paralysis or numbness or weakness in arms or legs lasting a few minutes—to paralysis for an hour or more. They can cause speech problems or visual difficulties, such as double vision or spots before the eyes. There can also be dizziness, confusion, falls, "blackouts," or fainting. Although these little strokes clear up spontaneously, they should be reported to the doctor for treatment and preventive measures, since the damage they cause can build up and lead to the symptoms of mental impairment.

When a diagnosis of multi-infarct dementia has been confirmed by a physician, the medical treatment will be different from that for Alzheimer's disease. In terms of dealing with the symptoms, however, the tasks of the family members involved are similar. Although the changes in behavior that these conditions cause will vary from person to person, the patterns and types of problems presented are the same.

Massive Strokes

The chronic mental impairment that results from multi-infarct dementia should not be confused with the damage caused by a massive stroke. A major stroke can cause loss of speech, comprehension, and vision, as well as paralysis and emotional instability, to name some of the most significant and disturbing symptoms. It can be transitory, with mild symptoms, or severe, with permanent disability. A major stroke can even cause death. It always causes a devastating crisis in the family.

Special rehabilitation therapy can often help to restore function of the paralyzed parts of the body, however, and speech therapy can help patients with aphasia to regain their ability to speak and to improve their ability to understand speech. The family can be taught rehabilitative techniques by the therapist, to speed up and maximize the recovery process. If you need to learn more about stroke, there is a book by Arthur S. Freese entitled *Stroke: The New Hope and the New Help*, which will give you a thorough understanding of the disease and its treatment.

I want to stress, however, that a stroke is unpredictable; there's a strong possibility of complete recovery in some cases and severe chronic disability in others. When the symptoms include mental changes, which often occur—whether temporary and reversible, or long-term and chronic—the family is confronted with the same challenge in understanding and coping with the behavior that results, as in multi-infarct dementia. The families of stroke patients will recognize many of the situations described in chapters 6 and 7, and can work toward solving problems more rationally.

Emotional instability and tearfulness are frequent

symptoms of stroke, which are particularly difficult for caring families to deal with. Depression, which often results from a stroke, can present its own symptoms of mental deterioration. The section on pseudodementia due to depression is very important for the family dealing with stroke.

Parkinson's Disease

Another condition that causes mental impairment and emotional symptoms in the aged is Parkinson's disease. Parkinson's disease has been known for over two hundred years as a nervous-system disorder that results in what was formerly called "shaking palsy." It is more accurately called a syndrome, or group of symptoms that appear together, whose cause, like Alzheimer's disease, is unknown.

Patients suffering from this disorder develop muscle rigidity, with uncontrolled tremors and a shuffling way of walking while stooped forward. When facial muscles stiffen, patients seem to stare, and as the muscles become unable to clear oral secretions, saliva accumulates and results in drooling.

These characteristics can give a patient a demented appearance, but historically mental impairment was not considered a significant part of Parkinsonism. Only in recent years has it been recognized that mental impairment can be linked to Parkinsonism, with studies showing that 20 to 80 percent of all Parkinson's patients experience mental deterioration. Mental impairment associated with Parkinson's disease seems to occur more in older patients, whose Parkinsonism developed late in life.

In Parkinson's disease, a specific part of the brain

shows damage, and there is a decrease of the neurotransmitter *dopamine* in many parts of the brain. With the revolutionary drug Levodopa (L-Dopa), which increases the dopamine in the body, many of the symptoms of Parkinsonism are relieved. Where mental impairment is part of the syndrome, however, L-Dopa seems to be less effective, and the symptoms progress more rapidly.

Although the relationship between Parkinsonism and mental impairment is unknown, there is clearly an association in a very large number of cases. If there is a Parkinson's patient in your family, you must learn to identify the signs of mental impairment and prepare yourself for the mental and physical changes that will occur: moderate to severe forgetfulness and confusion, disorientation, loss of understanding, emotional changes, and all of the other symptoms described in the previous chapter. Only by learning to recognize these changes as *symptoms* can you work toward acceptance of them as beyond the control of your relative. As your relative's mental condition changes him into a different person, your task in handling your feelings is the same as that of any other family going through this problem, regardless of the cause of the condition.

PSEUDODEMENTIA

A very important but often unrecognized or misunderstood possible cause of mental impairment in old age is the effect of depressive illness.

Depression is a common ailment, and it affects people of all ages. Some of the typical complaints expressed are feelings of sadness from which the person cannot be distracted, lack of concentration, loss of appetite, sleeplessness, and diminished interest in anything. When depression occurs in an older person, sometimes it is accompanied by forgetfulness, confusion, disorientation, and disordered thinking. When this happens, depression mimics dementia, because the symptoms are so similar. This is what is meant by the diagnosis "pseudodementia due to depression."

Although this is called *pseudo*dementia, the dementia symptoms are very real. The confusion and disordered thought processes have the same consequences as the dementia caused by Alzheimer's disease or stroke damage, and are just as difficult for the family. If the depression is not recognized and treated, the dementia symptoms can develop into an irreversible mental impairment. If the depression is treated, however, the dementia symptoms can improve, and the older person can be restored to normal functioning.

The study and treatment of depression has made most of its advances just in the past few decades since mood-altering drugs were discovered. As the neurotransmitter acetylcholine seems to be involved with memory and the speed of mental responsiveness, some neurotransmitters, particularly norepinephrine, are involved with our moods. A decrease in the amount of norepinephrine, which can be caused by many factors, is related to feelings of depression. Scientists believe that these neurotransmitters are also involved in other mental activities, such as memory and learning. Therefore, if an older person has lost a large number of brain cells as part of normal aging, it is possible that when something lowers the level of norepinephrine, his marginal level of functioning may be thrown off balance, leading to problems with thought processes in addition to depression. If the depression responds to treatment when the norepinephrine is increased, the older person's mental ability may improve as well.

Depressions have always been described as either *endogenous* (usually caused by something physical within the person), or *reactive* (caused by social and psychological factors). Most depressions are a combination of both types, since they are usually caused by some outside event, but how the individual reacts to the event is influenced by his personality and physiology. This involves several factors: (1) his health as determined by heredity, (2) his nutrition, (3) his life-style, (4) his metabolism, and (5) his glands, as well as the total effect of these variables on how his brain functions.

If you recognize this complexity, you can understand why, although depression is a very common problem, its cause is often unidentified.

Identifying Depression

Family members can play a significant role in identifying depression in a mentally impaired older person. First, there are so many outside events that can lead to normal depressive feelings in old age that the physiological connections are often overlooked. Some of the most common experiences that provoke depression in the later years are (1) difficulties in adjusting to retirement, (2) widowhood, (3) loneliness due to loss of relatives and friends, (4) serious illness, (5) loss of sight or hearing, and (6) fear of mental decline. Any of these experiences can trigger a physiological chain of events leading to a decrease in norepinephrine and malfunction of other enzymes. This deepens the depressive feelings and can tip the balance for the vulnerable older patient, adding symptoms of dementia to depression.

In addition to the social and psychological factors that can cause depressive feelings in old age, there is a known physiological change that may account for the increase in depressive reactions. An enzyme called monoamine oxidase (MAO) breaks down the action of neurotransmitters such as norepinephrine. Since monoamine oxidase normally increases with age, it may play a major role in decreasing the amount of norepinephrine in the brain of the older person, thereby making the older person more vulnerable to a depressive reaction to events with which he might have been able to cope earlier in life.

What often happens in these cases is that all efforts are made to help the older person overcome his depression by positive thinking and logic. "It could be worse" arguments abound, with countless examples of other people in the same or worse situations who were able to overcome their losses. What is overlooked is the *physiological* reaction to the psychological impact, a reaction that might respond to drug treatment and that could then enable the depressed older person to respond to talking things out.

Why should you have to be so alert to the physical and psychological components of depression that can be related to the other symptoms of dementia? Isn't it up to the doctors to recognize the causes of a physical or mental condition? Wouldn't it be presumptuous for you to raise so many questions when you bring your relative to a doctor for treatment?

Unfortunately, many doctors are ignorant of the latest knowledge in the field of aging. They may not have been trained to treat people in the extra ten or fifteen years that have been added to our life expectancy. Very few have ever had a course in geriatrics. Many are prejudiced about old people, treating most of their complaints as chronic and hopeless. "What do you expect at his age?" is an all-too-common response from the physician.

It is this attitude that can lead to a diagnosis of "senility" or Alzheimer's disease, with no attempt at treatment, when a depressed older person showing symptoms of confusion and listlessness or agitation, unable to handle mental challenges, is taken to a doctor. This is where your role is most important, first in trying to locate a doctor who is knowledgeable about problems of the aging and really interested in treating an older patient, and, second, in making the doctor aware that the problem is not chronic, by describing the patient's mental status prior to the onset of the problem.

Next, you must be aware that even doctors who have sympathetic feelings for their aged patients may not be capable of differentiating depression from the symptoms of dementia. It is known that in England and Canada, for example, there are many more admissions of the elderly to institutions for treatment of mental impairment where "depression" is the main diagnosis, rather than "dementia," the latter being more common in the United States. This has been attributed more to a negative attitude on the part of the American doctors toward the aging patient than to a greater tendency toward depression of elderly patients in England and Canada.

This diagnostic problem can also arise from difficulties in obtaining a thorough social and medical history. It is up to the family, therefore, if the doctor does not recognize the significance of depression as a factor in the appearance of other mental symptoms, to emphasize the development of the depressive symptoms and to describe the mental functions prior to the events precipitating depression.

It is important for you to be aware also that although some doctors prescribe too many medications too quickly, some doctors hesitate too long to prescribe medications for their older patients because of the possibility of multiple complications and side effects. Chapter 9 discusses the issues and dilemmas involved in medicating older people; at this point it is important to know that because of potential side effects, *medication to treat depression in an older person is often avoided even when it might lead to dramatic improvement.*

Other Causes of Depression

Depression can also be related to *nutritional deficiencies, drug reactions,* and *hormonal changes.* These possibilities should always be explored as part of a thorough medical investigation, which you must insist on. Don't be put off by the busy doctor who doesn't want to give time to a case that seems chronic and irreversible. Your relative should have the right to an exhaustive diagnosis; every possible cause should be ruled out.

Antidepressants

I believe that a significant proportion of old people would improve in all their mental functions if they were treated appropriately for depression. Appropriate treatment might require several trials of different medications of varying strengths, and may take weeks. This gives you an idea why this does not happen very often, for unless the older person has some concerned relative or friend nearby to monitor the process, or unless he has the means to pay for supervision, with frequent reports back to the physician on the effects of the drugs, a brief trial of antidepressants may not work.

When it is not practical for an older person to be supervised so closely, a period of treatment in a hospital may be effective. This can be very difficult to accomplish when the older person's mental state makes him uncooperative, or when the doctor is unwilling to suggest using the costly resources of a hospital for what appears to be an irreversible condition. Getting the depressed older person who needs that level of supervised treatment into a hospital may seem like an insurmountable task for the family, but it can be done if enough facts are provided to the physician, preferably a psychiatrist experienced with the aged.

Electroshock Therapy

Sometimes the depression and other mental changes are so severe that medications are ineffective, but electroshock therapy may help. In the medical community and among the public at large, there are very strong feelings against electroshock, but this is a relatively safe, painless process, well tolerated by the older patient. Although there is some memory loss immediately after treatment, this clears up, particularly if the electroshock is applied to the non-dominant part of the brain (the right side of the brain if the person is right-handed, and vice versa).

If the electroshock therapy is effective, and if the prior mental loss was related to the depressive illness, the patient's cognitive abilities might improve markedly.

Final Thoughts on Depression

It is not my intention to instill false hopes in families whose relatives suffer from mental impairment due to causes other than depression. It is my intent only to alert you to the possibility that *if* the symptoms of severe forgetfulness and confusion and other mental disorders are related to depression, they might clear up if the depression is treated. On the other hand, if the older person's depression is a reaction to his awareness of his mental losses, treating the depression will not relieve the other symptoms of mental impairment. The depression should still be treated, however, in order to lift the mood of the older person or relieve his agitation.

OTHER CAUSES OF PSEUDODEMENTIA

The previous section has discussed depression as the major cause of pseudodementia, since that is the illness most frequently associated with this condition. However, there are many other conditions that cause the symptoms of pseudodementia, which we can also call an acute or reversible organic brain syndrome. Remember, in medical terms, *acute* refers to a condition of *sudden* onset that is presumed to run a short course. If you bring your relative to a doctor with complaints of mental impairment that has started or worsened fairly suddenly, be sure to ask what may have caused this apparently acute condition. Your use of the term *acute* in your question to the doctor may encourage a more thorough investigation than if he assumes that your relative has a chronic mental impairment.

There are also many conditions that are reversible, although the symptoms seem to develop gradually, almost unnoticed at first. This section will cover the most frequent causes of mental impairment in which the family can play a significant role in diagnosis.

Any condition that causes a decrease in the amount of

oxygen available to the brain can cause mental impairment to an older person who is functioning with a marginal number of brain cells and a central nervous system that has slowed down somewhat in the normal course of aging. A special diagnostic problem in identifying the possible cause of the decrease in oxygen in an old person is that the usual symptoms may not show up. Even a heart attack might not be recognized in an older person, since he may not have the typical symptoms of chest pain and shortness of breath, and instead may suddenly become confused and disoriented.

Pneumonia, the common problem of urinary tract infection, high temperature, dehydration, drug intoxication, liver or kidney malfunction, anemia, or an electrolyte imbalance, all of which can show up in laboratory blood tests, are examples of possible causes of pseudodementia. Doctors are also usually alert to the possibility of thyroid dysfunction, a frequent cause of mental impairment, and one that can be reversed when the patient is treated. Therefore, it is urgent to get your relative to a good doctor quickly.

Malnutrition

A very frequent cause of pseudodementia is malnutrition. Lack of essential nutrients can be a direct cause of mental impairment, but it is easy to overlook. An older person who is not eating adequately, or not absorbing his food normally, may develop a zinc deficiency, for instance, and this may produce symptoms of mental confusion and memory loss.

A deficiency in calcium and/or magnesium, which is not uncommon, particularly in an older person who is not eating or absorbing his food adequately, can lead to depression or other symptoms of mental impairment by directly affecting the biochemistry of the body. These deficiencies do not always show up in the blood tests run as part of a routine medical workup. If there is reason to suspect a calcium or magnesium deficiency, study the older person's diet and try adding vitamin and mineral supplements.

Doctors often act as though vitamin and mineral therapy is a lot of hocus-pocus, or just another way to get the public to spend money unnecessarily. The frequent attitude expressed is "All you need is a balanced diet," which does not take into account that many older people do not eat a balanced diet, and even those who do may not be absorbing the nutrients because of the changes in their metabolisms. If you feel your doctor is too negative about the possible benefits of these supplements and there are no medical problems that would rule against taking them, you might try to get your relative to take them—along with an improved diet. There are many good books on nutrition that might help you in determining—preferably with the aid of a doctor or nurse interested in nutrition—what may be missing in your relative's diet and how to compensate for it. I've included three that I've found helpful in the section on recommended reading at the end of this book.

Consider the following possibilities in relation to your kin:

Loneliness. Many people do not enjoy eating alone. They may not feel like preparing regular, balanced meals for themselves. Even opening a can of food or heating a frozen dinner may be too much for the lonely older person. He may prefer tea and toast or coffee and doughnuts.

Nutrition programs that offer a hot meal in a social setting have been lifesavers for countless lonely old people, but sometimes it's difficult for the older person to get to the place where the meals are served. Perhaps transportation is not available. A fractured hip or leg might make it more difficult to get around. A fractured arm might make it too difficult to get dressed. Weather conditions might keep the older person at home, or impaired vision might make him fearful about going out alone. Impaired hearing might make him self-conscious about being with others or take away from the enjoyment of socializing with others. Increasing forgetfulness might also lead to self-consciousness. Urinary frequency or incontinence might keep an older person at home.

Many people don't like the idea of going to a nutrition program in the first place. They may feel it is taking charity, or they assume that they will not like the kind of people they'll meet there. They may say that they prefer to eat alone, even though they do not eat adequately.

Decreased Mobility. Any physical handicap can make it difficult for the older person to get out to shop for food, so any kind of fracture can lead to a change in eating habits. And the common problem of pain from arthritis can also make it more difficult to get out to shop. If the older person is too proud to ask for help or doesn't order food delivered to his home, it may be the beginning of a change in eating habits.

Decreasing energy. An older person may become frail or may experience a decrease of energy for various reasons, which might also make it more difficult to shop for food. Additionally, this loss of energy might make it too difficult to cook and clean up after cooking and eating, leading once again to the possibility of a tea-and-toast diet.

Inadequate income. An older person whose income does not keep up with rising costs may not be able to purchase the kinds of food he enjoys and is accustomed to. He may not be knowledgeable enough about nutrition to substitute less expensive foods to supply needed vitamins and minerals.

Ill-fitting dentures. If an older person has lost weight, his dentures may no longer fit comfortably, leading to serious changes in eating habits.

Loss of appetite. Sometimes an older person stops eating adequately because of a loss of appetite. This can be caused by many things, including medications and changes in brain function in the part of the brain that controls appetite. Or the older person may not even notice that he is hungry or thirsty.

Unbalanced diet. Persons also gain weight on unbalanced diets—with an excess of sweets and starches, for example. Overweight does not eliminate the possibility of malnutrition.

Medical diet. If a medical diet—such as low-salt, low-fat, or diabetic—is ordered, an older person may stop eating adequately because he no longer enjoys the food he is permitted.

Change in sense of taste. When an older person has lost a significant number of taste buds or his sense of smell, food may no longer taste good to him. Food may taste bland or bitter or sour, and he may not want to eat it.

Use of alcohol. Even a regular drink or two can cause a depletion of the B vitamins that are essential to the healthy function of the nervous sytem, and therefore to brain function.

Weight-loss diet. Finally, at times an older person gains weight because of lack of exercise, or slowed-down metabolism, or even from overeating due to boredom. In trying to lose this excess weight he may not eat a balanced diet. He may suffer from malnutrition, even though he's overweight.

The family must be sensitive and skillful in trying to determine whether any of these factors are relevant to their kin's situation. It is not always easy to get information from an older person, but the family should be alert to the possibility that any of these things may be affecting the mental change in their relative.

MEDICATION PROBLEMS

Because of the multiple problems that arise with advanced years, there is a strong probability that an older person takes a variety of medications. Such conditions as high blood pressure, heart disease, diabetes, arthritis, insomnia, nervousness, stomach distress, anxiety, and so on constitute only a partial list, and they can lead to an impressive array of drugs in the medicine chest.

Very often these medications are continued for years, without concern for what side effects might be occurring. Sometimes an older person goes to more than one doctor, looking for relief from persistent problems, and each doctor may prescribe different medication; a drug may unknowingly be added that will have an adverse interaction with the others. Some of these interactions might lead to symptoms of mental impairment.

The family should be aware that as the physiology of an older person changes with age, so does his reaction to drugs. Liver and kidney function decline even in the healthy elderly, requiring smaller dosages than are generally prescribed for younger people. The absorption as well as the distribution or transportation of a given drug is related to the circulatory system. Drugs can build up in an older person, stored in body fat, if the liver is not functioning properly or if the kidneys are not excreting adequately or if the older person's metabolism is not normal. A buildup of drugs in the system can be toxic, causing confusional states. If this occurs in an older person who has become somewhat forgetful, it is very easy for a misdiagnosis of senile dementia to be made.

MONITORING

It is also common for a toxic state to develop in the older person with a poor memory who takes his own medications. It is not always easy to arrange for supervision of medications when the older person lives in the community, especially since the family usually wants to help the older person maintain his independence. Sometimes it doesn't even occur to families to offer to help with medications. But if you want to prevent the possibility of mental impairment in your relative due to drug toxicity, you must monitor his medications, being aware of which ones he is taking and when he should be taking them.

I want to emphasize that you can be a natural partner with the health professional in the obvious need for monitoring medications for your forgetful older relative. All efforts must be made to overcome your relative's resistance if he insists that he is capable of self-medication, though you must understand his resentment of the seeming intrusion into his private life.

Adding to the difficulties of the forgetful old person

who is presumed capable of taking his medications safely is the fact that instructions on how to take them are often unclear. The old person, particularly if worried about his health, may not hear the instructions correctly in the first place, or he may forget them by the time he gets home. If he is taking several medications a number of times a day, the problem of remembering the instructions is compounded. Furthermore, the instructions typed on the label of the medication container might be too small for an old person with diminished vision. Or the written instructions might not be clear enough—does "take three times a day" mean before meals, after meals, or with meals? And how many people know that some medications should be taken on an empty stomach, which means one hour before meals or two hours after meals?

The family of the forgetful older person must be prepared to assume a protective role by checking with the physician and the pharmacist on the exact details of the medication regimen prescribed for their relative. Learn to ask what possible side effects to look for. Ask as well how long the old person should take the medications before being checked again by the doctor.

SIDE EFFECTS

Some of the most common medications that may lead to problems in your relative are those taken for hypertension (high blood pressure), anxiety (nervousness), depression, and sleeping complaints. If the dosages are monitored to meet the individual physiology of the vulnerable older person, and possible side effects are anticipated and reported back to the doctor for careful modification of the dosage, these medications can be very helpful. When symptoms of mental impairment appear, however, you should ask the doctor to check whether any of the medications, even if they have been taken safely for years, may now be responsible for these symptoms. (Some of the medications that can cause these symptoms are listed in Appendix 4.) Although doctors can usually identify the problem of drug intoxication when it is the cause of an acute mental impairment of sudden onset, it may be overlooked when it has developed gradually. A detailed drug history is the type of information an informed family or family surrogate must bring to the doctor to make an accurate diagnosis more feasible.

You must also be alert to the need for dietary supplements in relation to medication, such as the need for potassium when taking diuretics ("water pills"). Very often when a doctor prescribes a diuretic for a patient with high blood pressure or heart trouble, he advises the patient to drink orange juice or eat a banana. This is to guard against a diuretic-induced loss of potassium (which can cause symptoms of fatigue, apathy, and mental impairment). But your relative may not like orange juice or bananas, or he may not be able to buy them easily. You can learn of other sources of potassium—such as broccoli and carrots—which can make it easier for your relative to avoid the deficiency problems. A valuable tool in learning about medications and their effects is *The People's Pharmacy 2*, by Joe Graedon, an easy-to-read paperback.

Another common problem of which you should be aware is the extent of constipation as a complaint in old age, and the widespread use of laxatives. In addition to its being the result of a general slowing down of bodily function, constipation can be a side effect of many medications, such as drugs that are prescribed to relieve depression. It can also be a symptom of depression, and can cause confusion. Be sure to ask the doctor whether any medications should be changed or added with regard to these possibilities.

The laxatives that are taken to correct this problem can be a source of additional problems. In addition to generating dependency, many laxatives interfere with the absorption of essential vitamins and minerals, thereby leading to the possibility of mental impairment and nervous system disorders as well as countless other ills.

The forgetful, sometimes confused older person suffering from nervousness and possibly irritable behavior can take excessive doses of laxatives, and that makes the problem worse. Although this is a delicate and highly personal area, you can be helpful by trying to get as much information as possible, even by snooping around in the bathroom and bedroom to learn which laxatives, stool softeners, or enemas are being used by your relative. Present the facts to a doctor when bringing the older person for a visit. With this kind of information, which only a family member or close friend might be able to supply, the doctor is in a better position to advise appropriate treatment.

Be alert to changes in your relative's appearance, such as weight loss or gain, bruises of unknown origin, or different ways of walking or carrying himself. These physical changes may not be apparent to the doctor, but they may be significant in diagnosis. For example, falls or accidents that occur when no one is around may leave some bruises. The possibility of an accident might suggest an investigation of the possibility of a hemorrhage in the brain, which might in turn be responsible for changes in mental function.

If you are frustrated at this point about understanding the causes of mental impairment, don't despair. You are in good company. Just remember that there are many possible causes. By becoming knowledgeable about the multiple interrelated possibilities and learning to ask the right questions, you can assume a more effective role in determining whether your relative's condition is chronic or reversible.

For an extensive discussion of the many conditions that produce symptoms that can be misdiagnosed as chronic dementia, I would suggest an excellent book by Lawrence Galton: *The Truth About Senility and How to Avoid It* (see the list of recommended reading at the end of this book). The book deals with acute, reversible conditions, and it can be a valuable aid to the family who suspects that their relative's symptoms are related to a treatable condition.

4

The Crisis of Responsibility

Now that you've learned to recognize some of the symptoms and causes of mental impairment in your relative, let's take a look at why this condition is causing you so much pain. Obviously it hurts to witness the deterioration of someone you love. But why do you feel so overwhelmed?

We are all taught the biblical commandment to "honor thy father and mother" and to care for them in time of need; but how do you honor a parent whose mental impairment has robbed him of the ability to use a handkerchief when necessary or to know when to go to the bathroom? How do you handle your feelings when someone you looked up to and respected is no longer able to care for himself, let alone for you? How do you deal with your feelings of humiliation for the person who was? How do you accept the shock of seeing the person you revered and esteemed reduced to a state of near vegetation?

Each of us must struggle for his own resolution of these realities. It may be hard to honor the person who *is*, but it is still possible to honor the person who *was*, by concern and love and compassion for the transformed being who is now in a different level of existence.

One of the reasons that that you feel distraught is very likely that you are not really prepared to assume responsibility for your relative. Dealing with the problems of mental impairment calls for a whole new set of skills. You must learn how to assume a new role in relation to your loved one.

Taking on a new role toward your relative means changing customary ways of behaving, family patterns that may go back to your childhood. When your relative is no longer competent to care for himself, you must assume a protective role. When he becomes dependent upon you for basic maintenance and safety, you must be dependable. Most people are so unprepared to change their basic roles as sons or daughters, husbands or wives, "kid brothers" or "big sisters," that, when faced with this necessity, they are overcome with anxiety.

NEW ROLES

In the case of adult children of impaired parents, people sometimes talk of role reversal. When a parent can no longer care for himself, it is said that the child assumes the role of the parent. In most cases, however, this concept is not very helpful.

The very term *adult child*, which accompanies the concept of role reversal, indicates the ambiguities inherent in this new status. How can you be an adult and a child at the same time? Being an adult implies maturity; being a child implies an earlier stage of life and the need for guidance toward maturity. The use of the term *adult child* to describe the status of an increasing number of middle-aged persons whose parents are now living to old age only adds to the confusion surrounding the assumption of the new roles that are needed.

This problem with terminology also points up the inadequacy of the concept of role reversal to describe the tasks involved in your situation. Even though you may have to take on new responsibilities, as a parent would for a child, your emotional relationship with your parent or with a parent-figure does not change.

The role of child usually carries with it the need for parental approval. Throughout our lives, at some level we wish for our parents' approval and we feel guilty if we do something we think our parents wouldn't like. This is part of the conflict when we are forced to take responsibility for a parent, and especially when the parent is unable to accept us in this take-charge role. You can understand, then, how tempting it is, when an impaired but stubborn parent refuses your offered help, to retreat to an obedient-child role and do nothing.

On the other hand, when a child's needs must be met, the parent role does not carry with it the need for approval from the child. Parents often make decisions for children, even over their protests, when they feel it is in their best interests.

You can see how it might lead to upset and confused behavior if you are trying to assume an unrealistic parent role to your own parent.

THE FILIAL CRISIS

Margaret Blenkner, a leader in the field of aging and social work, identified a filial crisis that occurs in midlife if the elderly parents of an adult become dependent and the adult son or daughter must assume a protective role toward them. It is experienced as a crisis when sons and daughters are not able to change a pattern of looking up to the parent as an authority on whom they can depend for guidance and counsel. Even when this has not been the relationship in reality, it is often the ideal. And it is very painful to give up ideals.

In addition, there is a feeling of crisis when the parent first shows signs of needing care. It is so hard to know what to do and how to do it. No one wants to offend his parent by suggesting that that parent is not caring for himself adequately. And most older people insist that they are able to manage just fine, thank you! But the evidence of increasing frailty may be quite apparent.

Where is the role model for this new relationship? Middle-aged sons and daughters who are competent in managing most of the tasks in their lives find themselves uncertain as to how to assume a protective role and unsure about how much protection is needed. This is particularly the case when the parent denies the need for care.

PHYSICALLY FRAIL, MENTALLY CLEAR

This same uncertainty applies to families whose elders are mentally alert. Everyone goes through this dilemma if his parents survive to old age. Where parents are alert, however, the responsibility of the children is to offer help if it's needed but to allow as much independence as is desired or feasible.

Many families live in constant anxiety when an elderly relative becomes frail but refuses help. They worry that their relative will have an accident or suffer a heart attack and not be found until it is too late. For their own peace of mind they want their older relative to have help at home or to move where he will have supervision if it is needed.

If your older relative is able to acknowledge the risks but still refuses to accept help or to move, the issue becomes whether or not he is really alert and mentally competent. If so, he is entitled to his independence. Just as you insisted on your independence as you grew up, so you must acknowledge your relative's right to make independent choices, even to fail.

If the mental status of your relative is not clearly defined, however, and you are concerned about his judgment and his ability to make decisions, then professional help is needed.

MARITAL CRISIS

If your mentally impaired relative is your husband or wife, I know that you are going through an excruciatingly painful crisis as your partner slips away, leaving you frightened and bereft. Although what you are feeling cannot be compared to anything else, what I have discussed as part of resolving a filial crisis should be helpful to you as well. Whenever customary roles in a family can no longer be fulfilled because of illness, the roles must be changed. If your spouse becomes dependent, for example, you may have to assume a new and unanticipated role as protector or care-giver.

Some specialists have described this as the need to

take on a parenting role with your spouse. I feel that if you think you must assume a parenting role toward your husband or wife, it will only add to your difficulties and frustration. It is psychologically impossible for you to feel like a parent toward your spouse, even though many of your emotions may be similar to those of a loving, caring parent for a helpless child. Other feelings and needs remain that are part of the marital relationship, such as the needs for physical fulfillment and reciprocal caring, or the need to be proud of your spouse, which painfully remind you of your loss, even while your partner lives.

What is needed instead is a whole new set of roles. You need to assume the unfamiliar responsibilities involved in the role of protector, or care-giver, while adjusting to the loss of the role of partner, companion, and confidant.

FAMILIAL CRISIS

The same is true for brothers and sisters, aunts, uncles, nieces, and nephews who have to assume responsibility for any of their loved ones. The same sense of crisis can occur in the entire family, which is groping for cues, trying to figure out how to provide the care that is needed.

The moral obligation to take on a protective, responsible role toward your impaired relative is always experienced as a trauma if it is different from your former way of relating. In addition, some of the difficulties you are experiencing may be related directly to the personality of your relative and the quality of your past relationship. It is important to realize when taking on this new role that being dependable does not mean that you personally have to be the care-giver. Being responsible means making every reasonable effort to see that your relative is safe and getting proper care. I hope you realize by now that your confusion about protecting your relative is a very common response. The process of shifting or changing roles is typically experienced as a major family crisis. Some people are unable to act at all, while others may overreact. In some families, such a feeling of panic is generated that they are completely unable to cope. Old conflicts and jealousies sometimes resurface, interfering with sensible problem-solving.

FAMILY RELATIONS

Every family has its own style of relating and of assigning tasks and responsibilities. When you are faced with a family crisis, you may find that old resentments and hurts hover in the atmosphere, adding to the tension.

It's very important for everyone to realize that this is not the time to dredge up old problems. All of your energy is needed to sort out the facts, study the options, and work together toward deciding on the best course of action for your impaired relative.

In trying to deal with the new dependency of your relative, you may find that the old family patterns for assigning or assuming responsibilities don't work very well. The members of the family who could usually be counted on to shoulder all kinds of responsibilities may not live nearby and may not be able to take charge or even to share in direct care. Or if they do live nearby, they may not have the emotional or physical strength to assume responsibility.

If you are the only one in the same town as your dependent relative, you will feel resentful that the rest of the family is not exposed to the problem in the same way. You may feel put upon even while recognizing that the other members may also feel upset and frustrated that they are not living close enough to help. Or you may be angry, feeling that they wouldn't be helpful even if they lived in the same town.

For most of you, this is certainly not the first serious problem you've faced. You've managed to deal with other losses and disappointments, with other illnesses and crises. What makes this crisis different?

UNCHARTED TERRITORY

First, you are not prepared by instinct to know how to assume responsibility for a dependent older person. Nor is your general intelligence and sensitivity, no matter how high, sufficient to deal with the complex problems of your impaired relative. The need to assume these new roles represents a transition in your life for which there are no guides. You are in uncharted territory. Other transitions, such as becoming a student or getting married, are learned through role models in the family or community.

There are very few role models to whom you can look for guidance in your transition as care-giver or protector to your impaired relative. Since comparatively few people survived to very old age until recent times, there are few examples of how earlier generations coped with similar problems; where examples do exist, they are usually not applicable to your situation because of the social changes that have taken place during our lifetimes. For instance, the sister or brother who might have helped you with this problem probably lives in another city. Besides that, you are probably working full time, making it really difficult to be available to your relative.

What's more, because of advances in medicine, your relative can be expected to survive this illness for many more years than would have been possible during earlier generations. So you can see that for an extended period you will have to deal with very complex problems for which you have few guides and supports.

An important response to the absence of role models in the family is the recent development of support groups throughout the country, stimulated by the organization of the Alzheimer's Disease and Related Disorders Association. In 1975, when I first offered a training program for families going through these problems, there were no such programs or groups in the country. Now, because of growing awareness of the problem, groups are available in many cities. There, families can learn from one another and help one another through the long ordeal. (See chapter 12.) In years to come, the now uncharted world of the mentally impaired aged will become more familiar, but because of the unpredictability and uniqueness of each victim and his family, the tasks in coping will still sometimes be overwhelming.

GUILT

How much of yourself you feel you must give depends on how much of you is needed to bring together all possible resources. All family members should be called on to share responsibilities, with social services or institutions as a backup to family efforts. Don't be embarrassed to apply for social support services and for institutional care when they are indicated. You should know that these services were developed in response to needs for care that are beyond the capacity of the average family. Use of social services does not mean that a family is failing to care for its aged in time of need. You should continue to share in the care, however, along with the organizations now in place to meet these special needs.

Although all of this may seem logical to you, you may still feel guilty if you are not able to provide total care. If you do feel burdened by guilt, consider the following:

We measure ourselves against personal standards that may, however, need flexibility to accommodate changing times. Should we be harder on ourselves than we are on others? Have we set ideals for ourselves that are unrealistic and unattainable? Or are we too quick to forgive ourselves our shortcomings? Do we feel guilty because we fear that we have not lived up to our parents' expectations of us? But how do we know what our parents would have expected if they had foreseen the destructive force of mental impairment? We cannot know, yet the guilt is still there.

In one of my training groups there was a lengthy discussion about guilt. One member stated that Jews are more prone to guilt because the Jewish mother is particularly skilled at making children feel they are obliged to be dutiful through all eternity. A Catholic member argued against him, saying that the Catholic Church and the family, although forgiving of sins, made the devoted feel more guilty by setting very high standards for behavior. Another member, a Protestant minister, said, "You're both wrong. We Protestants invented guilt!" Clearly, guilt transcends all creeds.

Many people say they would not want their children to do for them what they are doing for their parents. This is an expression of the conflicts they must feel. While they do not want to pass on this ethic of caring for one's parents, they are unable to escape the burden of responsibility with a clear conscience.

How we behave toward someone in our family does not necessarily reflect how much we love him or whether we even like him. It reflects our sense of what we *should* do for him, which is dictated by our conscience. The social expectation of what is right to do for aged parents is now in the process of redefinition. But social rules for meeting the needs of the mentally impaired have not been formulated at all. The problems are still too new, too complex, and the options for meeting them are inadequate. It is no wonder that families who are confronted with these problems must grope for cues as to what is right to do and how to do it.

As your relative's condition demands more and more attention, you are caught up in a balancing act—trying to cope with these new problems for which you are not prepared, while meeting all of your customary responsibilities. And at the same time you may be feeling vulnerable yourself, perhaps anxious about your own future and what aging has in store for you.

To achieve a more comfortable balance between your many responsibilities and your personal needs, you must find your own answers to the following questions:

1. What does your relative need?
    a. How can those needs be met?
2. How much of yourself can you give?
    a. For how long?
    b. At whose expense?

The objective answer to how the needs can be met must take into account whether your relative is cooperative or not, and what resources and supports are available—such as finances or social-health services, numbers of helping relatives, quality of medical care, type of housing and community. This will put into perspective whether the amount and kind of care needed *can* be provided in your relative's home, in the home of someone in the family, or in an institution. But whether the care can be provided or not is largely dependent upon your relative's ability to cooperate, your family's ability to be persuasive as a unit, or your success in finding a physician who prescribes medication that can help your relative be more cooperative.

As to the question of how much of yourself you can give, you must first recognize the degree to which that will be influenced by your conscience, by how much you feel you *should* give, even while remaining aware of possible conflict and resentment. If you are tied to your parents or spouse by deep feelings of obligation, you will feel morally bound to do all in your power, and more, to meet their needs.

In some ways, the problems are greater in instances of mentally impaired spouses. If you are forced to institutionalize your spouse because the level of care needed clearly cannot be met otherwise, you are bound to feel tormented by feelings of self-reproach. There is a nagging feeling that your spouse has been abandoned even if he or she is receiving better care than at home. This is a normal response to a basic social ethic that dictates that you don't turn away from someone in trouble, and it is, of course, heightened by the words of the marriage ceremony. A frequently heard comment is "I couldn't live with myself if I did that."

Spouses often feel guilty even when providing care at home, especially if they are able to spend some time away from the problems. Yet taking time for separate activities is an important part of coping with the stress of living with someone who, though he may still seem very much the same physically, lingers between life and death.

Guilt and helplessness are the hallmarks of the transition you are going through: guilt about not finding a way to cure the condition; guilt about becoming impatient and irritable with your spouse's behavior; guilt about being angry with your spouse for not keeping his end of the marriage commitment; guilt about resenting the burden; guilt about looking ahead to the relief and freedom that will come with widowhood.

The relatives of elderly parents as well as the spouses of the mentally impaired must consciously work at resolving their guilt when it is unreasonable. By recognizing the source of some of your anxieties as coming from too rigid an adherence to ancient rules, you may be able to ease up on yourself. You must seek more flexible interpretations of some of the values that seem to cause irreconcilable conflicts between what you *want* to do and what you feel you *should* do. You must set realistic and achievable standards for yourself, or you will be condemning yourself to feelings of failure and worthlessness. But if you feel you should be doing more, do it!

I am not suggesting that you abandon ideals and basic values. Rather, I am trying to convey a sense of realism that may be needed to modify the demands of conscience. If your conscience makes you feel that you should save the world even though you know you can't, that's a "messiah complex." But if your conscience makes you sacrifice some of your own needs in order to feel better about your kin, it may be serving a useful purpose. Figure out how much you can give of yourself without unfair sacrifice of others you care about, and without pushing yourself to the point of resentment.

Although this may seem to be preaching, it is presented with the understanding that only you can work out what is best for you and your family. Even if you recognize that your behavior is not what you want it to be, you may not be able to change it, but you must still go on seeking your own solution. There are not clear-cut rights or wrongs in these situations. But as you review all of the examples and consider the issues, I hope that some new insights will help you in working through your problems.

ACCEPTING WHAT CANNOT BE CHANGED

I have found in my years of working with families that one of the most difficult problems is learning to accept the fact that this condition is chronic, that it will go on for years, and that it will probably get worse. All of us would like to believe that there is some way of treating brain damage so that its victims will improve. We don't want to feel that anything is hopeless. Many of us have been taught to believe in such maxims as "mind over matter" and "where there's a will there's a way," but no amount of positive thinking or wishing can will away chronic mental impairment and the changes in behavior and personality that follow. Even though you may emotionally need to deny the extent of your relative's impairment, it is necessary for you to recognize this as a first step in coping.

Everyone going through a terrible loss—through death or anticipated death or the loss of sight or a limb—

reacts first with shock and denial. There is a need to deny the problem until you have time to get used to it, gradually, in stages. It is a transition you go through while working toward accepting the unacceptable.

However painful it is to face and accept your loved one's mental condition, accept it you must. The hope that I can offer is that you will eventually learn to deal with these problems with more confidence, even though the pain is still there, as you acquire the knowledge needed to anticipate and assess your relative's behavior and to train yourself in more effective responses. With a deeper and broader understanding of your relative's symptoms, you will be able to face the illness realistically and gain better control over your reactions.

There is a well-known prayer (attributed to Saint Francis of Assisi) that has been adopted as the motto of the successful Alcoholics Anonymous program: "Grant me the serenity to accept what cannot be changed, the courage to change what can be changed, and the wisdom to know the difference." This motto has also been helpful in the training programs I have run for families of the mentally impaired aged, and it should be helpful to you as well, as you consider the problems we discuss and apply them to your own family situation. The task of accepting what cannot be changed is a fundamental challenge, and it will go on for the duration of your relative's illness, and even after.

CHANGING WHAT CAN BE CHANGED

Finding the courage to change what can be changed comes more easily to some than others. The nature of your relationship with your impaired relative from the pre-illness period will affect your courage. But you must develop the capacity to change what can be changed, just as you must acquire the wisdom to know the difference.

What are the most common and difficult problems that face you? These depend on whether your relative is your spouse, your mother or father, or other loved one, and whether he or she lives alone, with you or another family member, or in an institution. In the next chapters we will examine examples that represent a wide range of situations, with some suggestions and discussion following each. Although many of the case examples may not seem to apply directly to your family, reading through all of them will help you acquire a set of principles based on an understanding of the complexities involved. These principles will guide you when you are struggling with difficult decisions.

I once read that knowledge is what's left after you've forgotten the facts. I hope that after you have considered all of the cases and all of the issues, although you will forget many of the facts, you will be armed with a quality of understanding that will sustain you in your struggle.

5

The Diagnosis

*I*f you suspect that one of your relatives is mentally impaired, the first thing you must do is get a proper diagnosis. As the close relative or friend of a mentally impaired old person, you must take an active role in studying his behavior and share this information with a physician who is knowledgeable about problems of the aging. With the accurate information that only you can gather, and with the new diagnostic techniques available, the physician can determine whether your relative has an acute or chronic mental impairment, and can prescribe appropriate treatment. If it is a chronic progressive illness, you must be sure that there has been a distinction made in diagnosing as to whether it is senile dementia of the Alzheimer's type, multi-infarct dementia, or another form of mental impairment, since treatment of each will be different.

With your awareness of the meaning of these terms and of the professional attitudes associated with the probable course of the illness, you can become an effective partner in the care of your loved one by assuming an advocate role on his behalf as a first step in accurate diagnosis.

How do you know if and when to intervene? This is where professional guidance is essential. A thorough medical workup is always the first step, preferably by a physician who is knowledgeable about the problems of older people.

But finding good medical help to do a proper diagnostic workup is often a very difficult problem for the caring family. If you have not yet overcome this obstacle, I will outline here the steps you can take toward this goal.

THE WORKUP

First, if your relative is known to a doctor, discuss your observations and concerns with him. Find out which drugs have been prescribed and try to determine for yourself whether they have been taken properly. This information is essential for an accurate diagnosis, but is often ignored because of the difficulty in getting the facts. Uncovering the facts about your relative's medication sometimes calls for the skills of a detective, checking for dates of prescriptions and counting the number of tablets in the bottles. This can be a terrible hurdle if your relative resents your intrusion into such private matters, but you must try to handle the situation calmly, with a matter-of-fact approach. Explain to your relative the importance of telling the doctor exactly how many medications are taken, including nonprescription medications, in order for him to get proper treatment. Try to get your relative's help in locating all of the drugs in the house, but if he cannot help, inspect the medicine cabinet, dresser drawers, night tables, kitchen cabinets, refrigerator, clothing pockets, pocketbooks, and any other areas where medication might be. I know that it is easier to tell you to handle this task calmly, with a matter-of-fact approach, than it is to do it. But it is such an important part of the process of providing the doctor with an accurate history that you should do everything in your power to succeed.

It is difficult to stay calm if your relative is upset, so you may find it helpful to rehearse what you might say if he gets excited and angry. Try to imagine what he might say and how you would respond to be reassuring. You might even play out the scene with a friend or another relative to prepare yourself for the encounter. It might not be anything like what you will go through, but then again, it may be very helpful.

BEING CAUGHT IN THE ACT

Try to understand your emotions at this stage. Most of the family members I have worked with became very upset when they had to take charge in such personal areas. If you are upset too, it may be because you are reminded of other times in your life when you had to become involved in situations that were very uncomfortable.

For instance, many people have had the experience of

being worried about whether their child was getting into something he or she shouldn't, such as smoking, taking drugs, or stealing. They may have been tempted to look through their child's belongings secretly. Or perhaps you are reminded of a time in your own adolescence when your parents discovered you doing something wrong. Such traumatic events often lie buried within us, and give no cause for any particular concern until the feelings are reactivated by an event that involves similar emotions. Probing into the private areas of your relative's life may provoke just such anxious, disturbed feelings. By recognizing the source of some of these strong emotions, you can more easily overcome them.

If you feel it is too difficult for you to become involved in such personal areas, you may find it helpful to call in a public health nurse to do an evaluation at home. Also, your relative may be less embarrassed to talk to a professional nurse. However, if your relative is convinced that he's managing well and doesn't need help, even the most experienced professional may not get any more information than you can. The most important thing is to try by every possible means to learn as much as you can about his habits.

RELATING TO THE DOCTOR

Now we come to the next problem: assuming an appropriate role in your relative's medical care. Even though you may want to discuss your relative's condition in detail with the doctor, your involvement may not be understood or welcomed by him.

Most doctors are taught in medical school that they

have full responsibility for diagnosing and treating their patients. By the time they graduate as physicians, they have had to develop complete confidence in their ability to assess and manage the complexities of the practice of medicine. They have been taught that successful treatment requires the confidence of the patient in the doctor, and this style of practice does not welcome many questions. Furthermore, doctors are usually very busy, and they don't allow much time for questions and discussion with patients and their families.

Many people feel like retreating at the first impatient response from the doctor. Most people don't want to feel as though they are being "pushy."

You may understandably ask yourself whether you really have to be aware of all the physical and psychological possibilities that might affect your relative. You may feel that it's up to the doctor to recognize all of the possible causes of a physical or mental condition. You may even feel that you have no right to raise so many questions when you bring your relative for evaluation and treatment.

While you may feel uncomfortable raising questions with a doctor who does not seem happy to help you in your efforts, your success in this matter could be critical for your relative. Many doctors are unfamiliar with the latest knowledge in the field of aging. Even many of those with a large practice among the aging have never had a course in geriatrics, which would help them understand the complexities of the older patient. Very many prejudge the elderly and view most of their complaints as chronic and hopeless. "You'll have to learn to live with it" is what one often hears from the physician; this reflects the attitude that, rather than being symptoms of a specific condition or disease, most problems are normal for old age and therefore do not warrant treatment.

Often there is also an unspoken attitude: Is it worth my investing a lot of time and effort in an old person with a dubious prognosis? These are attitudes that can lead to a diagnosis of senility or Alzheimer's disease, with no attempt at diagnostic precision, when an old person is seen with various symptoms of mental impairment. This is where your ability to assume your rightful role with the doctor is most significant.

ISSUES TO RAISE

It is important for you to know that *many* of the medications which older people take for common problems—such as high blood pressure, heart conditions, or sleeping difficulties—can lead to symptoms of mental impairment. Sometimes these symptoms show up only after the person has been taking these drugs for years. And there are so many ways that they can accumulate in the elderly system that a busy doctor might not even start to investigate. For example, if the kidneys or liver are not functioning perfectly, the drugs may not be processed correctly, and mental symptoms might develop. If your relative is well on in years, however, the doctor may very easily accept these symptoms as part of the aging process and not consider the relationship to medications.

Ask the doctor whether any of the medications, or combinations of the medications, might have side effects that cause confusion or other mental symptoms. Then ask whether any of these medications could cause these symptoms if they have built up in the system. If the doctor finds your specific questions too probing and answers you brusquely, be tactful, but point out that since your relative is not capable of managing for himself, you must now assume responsibility. Try to enlist the doctor's cooperation by pointing out that there are many areas with which you are unfamiliar, such as your relative's medication regime, and you need his help in making sure that you are doing everything possible for your relative's protection. Tell him that you read about these possibilities in a book dealing with this specialty, and that you want to be sure your relative's current problems are not caused by medications.

The doctor will probably do a physical examination and order a series of blood tests to check on whether the mental changes are related to specific physical conditions. Remember, a previous chapter detailed the many illnesses that could cause mental deterioration: heart conditions, anemia, thyroid problems, and liver or kidney disorders were a few examples. At this stage, if your relative is fortunate enough to have a reversible condition, your ability to help in obtaining an accurate diagnosis might make the difference between treatment and neglect, between life and a living death.

Before a diagnosis of Alzheimer's disease or other chronic mental condition is made, the doctor will order other tests, such as the CAT scan and electroencephalogram. These tests, which provide pictures of the brain and brain activity, are painless, but be prepared for the possibility of frightened reactions. Most of the personnel working with the aged are quite skilled in reassuring the patients and getting them through the process, but you may be called upon for extra encouragement.

If your relative's doctor has not been helpful in this stage of your problem, you should proceed as though your relative had no doctor available, and begin to investigate another source of medical assistance.

WHEN YOUR RELATIVE HAS NO DOCTOR

I would suggest first contacting the Alzheimer's Disease and Related Disorders Association through their toll-free telephone number (see Appendix 3). When you reach them, ask for the telephone number of the chapter nearest to where you live. When you contact your local chapter, you will find them very helpful in sharing information about all kinds of resources, including the names of local physicians who are especially interested in problems of mental impairment. This contact can be a shortcut in what otherwise may be a difficult process.

If for some reason you cannot get this information through an ADRDA chapter, you will have to use your ingenuity in locating the best specialist. Ideally this would be a geriatrician, a physician whose specialty is the medical care of the aged; however, there are very few doctors who have been trained in this new specialty. A family medicine specialist, an internist, or a neurologist would be appropriate to do the diagnostic workup. One way to start your search is to ask your own doctor for a referral, emphasizing the desirability of finding someone who is interested and experienced with the aged. If that does not turn up a concerned doctor, and if you have time to make a lot of phone calls or write letters, you might want to contact the following organization:

> American Geriatrics Society
> 10 Columbus Circle, Room 1470
> New York, NY 10019

Ask for a listing of medical members who are in your area. These doctors are not necessarily geriatricians, but they demonstrate their interest in geriatrics by their membership in this professional organization.

Sometimes, when the family is interested primarily in evaluating the judgment and competence of their relative, the most appropriate professional to contact might be a geriatric psychiatrist. I have found that psychiatrists who have specialized in this field are particularly sensitive to the many potential causes of mental impairment and are generally very helpful to the family.

The psychiatrist can assess the level of competence of the old person and recommend to the family whether it is safe for the relative to be alone or unsupervised. I would again suggest calling the Alzheimer's Disease and Related Disorders Association as a shortcut in locating a psychiatrist experienced with these problems. If the ADRDA cannot help you with this, and if you would like to get the name of some geriatric psychiatrists in your area, a membership list can be obtained from this organization:

American Association for Geriatric Psychiatry
230 North Michigan Avenue, Suite 2400
Chicago, IL 60601

The psychiatrist would suggest the route for further medical workup if he thinks it's necessary, and he would also probably suggest an assessment by a nurse and social worker to evaluate what help is needed for the safety and care of your relative. If your relative needs help but cannot recognize it, these professionals may be able to help you take charge. If your relative is still capable of independent living, this assessment can be very reassuring to you, but you will still need to be vigilant for changes in the future.

These suggestions for how to go about the difficult task of obtaining a proper diagnosis cannot possibly deal with the uniqueness of each and every situation. With the increasing membership and chapters of the Alzheimer's Disease and Related Disorders Association, many of you will find help with these practical issues. For the rest of you, I have prepared a guide to some of the agencies you can contact for help, depending on the financial status of your family. Please refer to Appendix 3.

THE SOCIAL WORKER

Most people have no experience with social workers and are uncertain about what they do. Many believe that social workers are primarily for poor people who need financial assistance. But the professional social worker is skilled in assessing the psychological and social problems of people regardless of their income level. The social worker is trained to help people resolve their emotional and practical problems, through better understanding of themselves, through developing better methods of coping, and through appropriate use of community resources and services.

By virtue of education and experience, a social worker is most suitable to help families of the mentally impaired aged. He can help sort out feelings and examine situations realistically, with knowledge of available resources and entitlements, and the expertise to cut through the red tape of the social and health care systems.

Unfortunately, there are very few such professionals with qualifications in geriatrics. If you live in a large city, you may find some social workers who are newly specialized in counseling the aged and their families, either on a private basis or through one of the many social service agencies available to help the elderly. See Appendix 3 for suggestions as to how to locate them.

If you take the time to make contact with a social worker who is knowledgeable about mental impairment in aging, you may find it a significant shortcut to resolving many of your problems.

When, after a thorough evaluation is completed, there is a definite diagnosis—of Alzheimer's disease or any other mental impairment—your continuing task is to resolve your filial crisis responsibly by learning to assume a protective role and finding the most appropriate way to provide care. If you have recently gone through the process of obtaining the diagnosis, I know that you must feel devastated by the confirmation of your worst fears. You must be wondering what will happen and how long this illness will go on. You may ask the doctor for a prognosis.

THE PROGNOSIS

Be prepared for the doctor to be very vague and general in his answer. Some years ago, doctors used to estimate that someone with Alzheimer's disease or other chronic deteriorating mental condition would live two to five years. Now, with better medical care, that estimate has been revised to three to ten or even fifteen years. But this is only a "guesstimate." There is no scientific basis for predicting the span of time in which the illness will run its course, or what other illnesses may come along to change the situation.

There is also no way of predicting which symptoms

will show up in each patient, or how severe these symptoms may become. Each family must constantly adjust to the changes that will occur in its impaired relative. However, through studying the typical problems presented in this book and considering the discussion as it may apply to your family situation now and in the future, you will be somewhat prepared for the difficulties ahead.

GENETICS

And a final word: One of the first questions that comes up after the diagnosis of Alzheimer's disease is verified is "What are my chances of getting it?" This is a natural concern of anyone whose blood relative has such a terrifying illness.

Let me reassure you that at present there is no evidence that you are at any great risk for developing Alzheimer's disease. A recent review of the literature on the subject found that no clear genetic course has been established. So put aside this fear and use all of your energy to deal with your relative's condition.

6

Case Studies: Problems in the Home

During my many years of practice with the aging, I've met lots of people and heard many stories. Everyone's is unique, but I have found some patterns that come up again and again.

Here are some cases that represent the problems facing many of you. The cases I have selected make no reference to race or ethnicity, although it is obvious that these significant identities are of great influence in how family problems are perceived and handled. I think that the following cases present most of the important problems you are facing, and I hope you will find that they transcend sectarian issues.

MRS. WELLS

Mrs. Wells, an eighty-five-year-old Philadelphia home-maker who was widowed twenty years ago, had adjusted to living alone, keeping busy with the ladies' group from her church, her senior citizen center, and her volunteer work at the nearby hospital. She prided herself on not being a burden to her children: a daughter, Betsy, who lived in the suburbs of Philadelphia, a son who lived in New York, and another daughter who lived in a retirement community in Florida. Mrs. Wells cherished her privacy, and she never entertained any ideas of giving up her comfortable, memento-filled apartment, even though her children often urged her to move into some kind of protective setting, particularly after she had turned eighty. She was satisfied with the amount of contact she maintained with her family in person and by telephone, at least once a week.

During the past few years, Mrs. Wells's family became aware that she was slowing down considerably. She complained about her memory, and was becoming very repetitious without being aware of it. Her failing vision made her less secure in the streets, and her diminishing hearing made it difficult for her to continue her volunteer activities and senior center attendance. As she moved around less, arthritic pain started to plague her. It became an ordeal even to get around in her apartment.

When it became difficult for her to manage her checkbook and pay her bills, she was relieved to have her son take over this responsibility. Since her income went directly into her checking account, all that had to be done was to have his name added to the account. She accepted his offer of help because she knew it was not too much for him to do. After all, there were very few bills to pay.

Since Betsy lived closest to her, it was natural that she take on the responsibility of shopping for her mother, preparing meals, and even cleaning the house. Recently, Betsy noticed that the food she prepared for her mother was not always eaten. Mrs. Wells insisted that she was eating regularly, but she was getting very thin.

For the past two months the family has been very upset. Mrs. Wells is neglecting her appearance, and she has become withdrawn. She dozes off in front of the TV most of the day. She no longer telephones anyone. The children have had several telephone conferences about what they should do for their mother.

Betsy's sister and brother are both critical of her even though she is the one who is doing the most for their mother. They feel she should insist that Mrs. Wells move into a nursing home. They are unhappy that being so far away makes it impossible for them to do anything more than give advice, but at the same time they blame Betsy for not having convinced their mother that she should move into an institution. Of course, Betsy is upset with their criticism and is beginning to feel dumped on. But she has never felt comfortable arguing with her older sister and brother.

They have decided that they should all share in the expense of a homemaker for Mrs. Wells, but Mrs. Wells has refused, insisting that she can take care of herself. Betsy was almost in tears when she pointed out that the kitchen floor was dirty and sticky. Mrs. Wells denied the obvious mess with the remark, "Don't be silly. You can eat off my floor."

Betsy, the youngest daughter, feels closest to her mother, but she is exhausting herself by trying to shop for her mother and clean her house at least once a week. She is now fifty-five herself and working full time as a secretary in a very busy law firm. She feels her mother should move in with her, but she is afraid that her husband might object. Instead, she has asked her son, a graduate student, to look in on his grandmother occasionally during the day when he has some free time. He was very upset when, in recent visits to her, she confused him with her son. Further evidence of her increasing confusion turned up when he opened the refrigerator for a cold drink and found his grandmother's heating pad and bedroom slippers.

To her family's pleas to accept help from a homemaker, Mrs. Wells replied, "Don't worry about me. I've lived long enough. I'm ready for the Good Lord to take me." The family feels completely helpless.

Discussion

What should Mrs. Wells's family do? What *can* they do?

It is obvious that Mrs. Wells is no longer capable of taking care of herself, nor does she have the judgment to recognize this. Mrs. Wells's family must now assume a responsible role and take some actions for her protection. However, if Mrs. Wells does not cooperate in some way, plans for her care can only be carried out tentatively and with difficulty.

As a first step, the family must see to it that Mrs. Wells is taken to a doctor for a medical workup. If Betsy can't get her to cooperate, the son should come from New York to take her to a doctor. Since she has trusted him to take care of her checking account, she will probably allow him to accompany her to the doctor.

Betsy must take care not to feel jealous of her mother's trusting relationship with her brother, since that will only add to the feelings of strain. She must learn to appreciate whatever help is given to share the burden of responsibility.

If Mrs. Wells still refuses, the family must wait awhile and try again. Sometimes the persistent efforts of a united family can break through the resistance of the older relative.

At the same time that Mrs. Wells's family is working on getting her to a doctor, they should move ahead with getting help for her at home. Since they have already agreed to share the cost of a homemaker, Betsy should go to a home-health agency to hire someone with special skills in handling the needs of a mentally impaired older person. This might be a home attendant or housekeeper with enough patience and sensitivity to provide care even to a resistant old person. The challenge to the provider of care to an unwilling recipient is to find some approach that communicates competence and concern.

Sometimes a matter-of-fact approach works. "I'm here to shop for you, prepare your meals, and see that you eat properly. Your daughter tells me you always liked to look nice. So we're going to make sure your clothing is cleaned, help you take your bath regularly, and wash and set your hair. I'll keep your house nice and clean, just the way you like it. When the weather is nice, we'll try to get outside for a little exercise."

This is an ideal model, however; unfortunately there are not always people available with the intelligence, personality, and originality to carry out this approach. Betsy can take on the role of trainer, to teach the attendant how to approach her mother.

At this stage of Mrs. Wells's decline, she probably would not have the energy to put up a fight. She might improve somewhat with regular meals, better nutrition, and supervision of medication for her arthritic pain. She might then protest again to her family that she doesn't need the help. They must maintain the position that she would get worse again if the help were discontinued and that she will need care for the rest of her life.

Most home-health agencies have a social worker or case manager to help the family assess needs and modify services as necessary. Betsy should contact the social worker and talk over the family's concerns so that the case manager can be prepared to assist them in their tasks.

The Prognosis

Since Mrs. Wells's condition came on gradually, over a period of several years, it is probable that her mental and physical status will continue to worsen over a period of several more years, even with the supervision of an excellent home attendant. At some point, she may require twenty-four-hour supervision if she doesn't sleep through the night.

The cost of this type of care might be too much of a burden over a long period of time, and the family may have to look into the matter of eligibility for help through Medicaid, which might supply this type of care if it can be documented that otherwise Mrs. Wells would be in a nursing home. For a discussion of practical issues concerning Medicaid applications, see chapter 10.

In addition to the financial problem of twenty-four-hour care from a home attendant, sometimes the family finds that the help available is not always reliable. They may face regular crises when someone in the family must stay with the patient because the attendant fails to show up. It is usually prudent for the family to explore the possibility of a nursing home admission for the future, as a backup to the care being provided at home. (See chapter 10 on nursing home admissions.)

Unless there is a great deal of money available for this type of care, involving at least two shifts of caretakers and substitutes for the days missed (for illness, family problems, or just the need for time off), the family may find that it is very difficult to manage for longer than several months. At current prices, this will cost at least $25,000 per year, not counting rent, utilities, food, and so forth. All the best intentions in the world may not make it possible for her family to keep Mrs. Wells at home if she takes years to die.

This sounds cruel and unfeeling, but it is important that it be said, because part of the anguish of the family of the mentally impaired aged person results from the fact that the physical self takes much longer to die than does the mental self.

Families very often feel guilty, as though they have failed to comply with the wishes of their loved ones, when their needs become too difficult to meet at home and they turn to a nursing home to take over. They hear about other families who say that their parent was allowed to die in the dignity of his own home. We have all heard the assertion that "I would never put my mother or father in a nursing home."

In response we must ask:

1. How long did the problem go on?
2. Was the person involved living alone?
3. Was he mentally impaired or just physically impaired?

4. How many relatives were available to share in the supervision of the care provided?
5. How much money was available for the care?

The answers to these questions will probably point up the fact that unless there are lots of relatives and/or lots of money, when the time comes for twenty-four-hour supervision of a severely mentally impaired old person, that level of care can usually be provided in the home only for a limited time.

Other Possibilities

Some families find it preferable to provide care by moving their relative into their home. This may work out under some circumstances.

The following questions may clarify some of the issues:

1. Does the care-giving relative have the emotional endurance to witness the decline of a loved one?
2. Is the older person mobile and in need of constant surveillance?
3. Is the older person quiet and passive, or restless, agitated, talkative, repetitious, argumentative?
4. Is the older person cooperative or obstructive? Frightened and clinging? Anxious and whining? Sad and withdrawn? Gentle and good-natured? Nervous and hostile?
5. Is the behavior consistent and predictable, or erratic and fluctuating?

6. How many relatives are available to share the burden?
7. Is there money available to pay for an aide so that the care-giver does not become overwhelmed and exhausted?
8. Are there members of the household who resent the inclusion of the mentally impaired person? If so, what effect does this have on the main care-giver and the other family members?

Reviewing these questions and considering their implications should indicate the potential pitfalls in moving the mentally impaired older person into the home of a relative.

Pharmacological Magic

There is an important aid in caring for an older person who may be difficult because of restlessness, agitation, and other irritating behaviors, or whose depressive behavior may seem to be contagious. If the older person's doctor can prescribe the right medication and the right dose, the difficult behavior can be relieved. Negative and unrealistic attitudes must be overcome in order to make use of the pharmacological interventions that can make both the older person and the care-giver more comfortable. The potential effect of medication is an important element in making decisions and taking action on behalf of the mentally impaired older person. This is a step that is often overlooked in the assessment stage, but it can be crucial in effecting the best plan for all concerned (see chapter 9).

Deciding Factors

How can Mrs. Wells's family know whether it will be better to keep her in her own home with help or move her into one of their homes? And will things get worse if they move her and it doesn't work out?

We really have no way of knowing. There are some who might say that the older person will be worse off if the move proves to be a failure and the older person has to be moved again. Some may say that the family will be worse off if they have failed to provide care for their loved one in their home, in which case they will feel both defeated and guilty.

In my practice, this has not been the experience of many families who try to provide this kind of care. If it doesn't work out and they must later arrange for institutional care, they usually feel that they did their best to meet their obligations to their impaired kin and they usually express less guilt than those families who have not tried this alternative.

Some people are more self-aware than others. They know themselves well enough to be able to predict how they will feel and react under most circumstances. They might be correct in anticipating their reactions to their impaired kin, and therefore might be able to avoid decisions with which they cannot live. Many others have less control over their emotions. They cannot easily predict what their reactions will be to the unsettling and often unpleasant behavior of their relatives. The latter group may be more dependent upon a trial-and-error approach to making decisions regarding their kin.

No one has the right or the ability to make a value judgment about these momentous decisions. And yet opinions are often expressed about what the family should or should not do. There are no right or wrong solutions— only tentative ones that may or may not work out for a given period of time.

Inaction

Thus far we have discussed what Mrs. Wells's family might do on her behalf, which we may summarize as follows:

1. Get medical assessment and follow up on any medications ordered.
2. Provide care in her own home.
3. Move her into the home of one of the children and provide care.
4. Arrange for nursing home admission.

There is another option. They might do nothing. If Mrs. Wells has the strength to resist their efforts on her behalf and throws out the home attendants they send in, they may feel there is nothing else they can do.

It is quite natural for the family to be very angry with a relative who is causing so much trouble. Doing nothing in the face of so much need may be a reaction to frustration and helplessness, or it may be understood as an act of passive aggression, an unspoken expression of anger. This happens more often than is realized, and sometimes it is the only course left. The family waits and worries until a crisis occurs that requires hospitalization, such as a fractured hip, or collapse from dehydration or malnutrition. When the impaired older person is forced into treatment by such circumstances, it is usually easier to make a plan for future care.

Beware, though, that the old person's home is not given up at this time. Often it is, under the assumption that this is in the best interest of the older person who was not able to accept care until this point. What is misunderstood is that it is sometimes possible for the impaired older person to accept the realistic need for care *after* a period of institutional treatment, and he might be able to function at home again with proper help, provided that the home hasn't been given up precipitously.

Commitment Proceedings

Another option—an alternative to doing nothing and waiting for a crisis—is to enlist the aid of a physician or health agency in order to have the person committed for treatment. If a psychiatrist feels that the older person is mentally incompetent to care for himself and is in danger of harming himself or others, the older person can be taken to a hospital for treatment, even against his will. This option is rarely exercised, however, because there are very strong feelings about forcing someone into treatment. This will be discussed further in chapter 7.

We have considered, in relation to Mrs. Wells, several serious problems that will be familiar to many of you. The questions raised should form the basis for the principle of tentative planning, with prepared alternatives in view of the uncertainty ahead.

Helplessness, Anger, and Guilt

The complex issues that have surfaced in the case of Mrs. Wells and her family will come up in many of the case examples that follow, but they will never be identical since each case presents the issues in a unique context. But the feelings of helplessness and anger in response to that helplessness will often be present. Then guilt is sure to creep in. Recognizing these normal reactions can help in cutting through the emotional tangles that interfere with rational problem-solving.

MR. AND MRS. BARNETT

Mrs. Barnett, an eighty-year-old former teacher, lives with her eighty-two-year-old husband. They've been married fifty-three years, and during that time they have never been separated. He is still working a few days a week as an accountant in the same firm he has served for forty years. He is very upset, however, by his wife's mental condition, which has been deteriorating for the past three or four years. They live in a three-room apartment in New York City at a modest rental in a middle-income, high-rise housing development.

As Mrs. Barnett became more and more confused, she was unable to accomplish even the most familiar household tasks. Mr. Barnett would leave her written reminders and instructions on when to peel the potatoes and wash the salad so that when he came home he would only have to put the chicken or steak on the broiler. He found that his wife could no longer understand the instructions, and often she turned the kitchen topsy-turvy trying to find something—but she wasn't sure what. When he stopped leaving assignments for her, Mrs. Barnett would telephone their daughter, who also lives in New York, and a son who lives in Connecticut, asking them what she was supposed to do. They tried to calm her down, but their reassurances were futile. Five or ten minutes later she would call again in a panic, sometimes dialing a wrong number. When their telephone bill came to over $500 one month, Mr. Barnett had a lock installed on the phone. This upset Mrs. Barnett terribly, as she couldn't understand the reason for the lock. She managed to break it twice. She became very agitated, even on the days when her husband was at home. Occasionally she would walk out of the apartment while he was reading. Once she wandered around until a neighbor recognized her and brought her home. Several times, she wandered in the hallways on different floors and disturbed other tenants by knocking on their doors, not knowing where she belonged. On one occasion the superintendent became very upset when she pressed the "stop" button on the elevator, trapping herself between floors. It took hours before the elevator service company came to rescue her, and when she was freed, she had messed up the elevator with urine and feces. Mr. Barnett was told that they would be evicted if he didn't put his wife in a nursing home.

Mr. Barnett had resisted getting a housekeeper to assist them, for two reasons. First, he was concerned about the cost, although he had managed to save a fair amount of money and had a comfortable income from social security and an annuity. He was so accustomed to living on a very modest budget that he could not easily bring himself to spend the amount needed for a full-time housekeeper. Second, they had a small apartment, and Mr. Barnett felt that it would interfere with his privacy to have an employee in the house all day long.

There were several family conferences after the superintendent threatened to evict them. Their daughter is devoted to her mother, but since she was recently divorced and is raising two young children alone, she is unable to do more than visit once a week or take her mother out with her once or twice a week. The son who lives in Connecticut has his own troubles—a wife who is suffering from what may be terminal cancer. Although they couldn't offer any help to their father, both children vehemently opposed his placing their mother in a nursing home. Despite their protests, Mr. Barnett decided to find a nursing home for his wife because he felt unable to handle the problem any longer. He himself was starting to have some physical complaints, and he felt that if his wife weren't placed in a nursing home, they would both "go down the drain."

In the process of exploring the possibility of admission to a nursing home, as part of the application procedure Mrs. Barnett was taken to a physician and a psychiatrist for examinations. She was found to be in good physical condition, and it was suggested that she take Haldol, a drug that is sometimes effective in treating agitated, confused patients. At the same time, Mr. Barnett was told that a nursing home placement would use up most of his savings; eventually he would be impoverished by his wife's nursing home costs. He then went out and hired a housekeeper who would cook, clean, and be a companion to Mrs. Barnett. After a few weeks, Mrs. Barnett responded very well to the Haldol, which eliminated her agitation and her need to make telephone calls and wander out restlessly.

The Barnetts have had a full-time housekeeper for two years now. She lives in at present, since Mrs. Barnett has kept waking up at night, not allowing her husband to get any rest. The housekeeper sleeps in the bedroom with Mrs. Barnett, and Mr. Barnett sleeps on the living room couch. He is very unhappy with the situation. He is physically frail, but he forces himself to continue working because he doesn't feel he has a place of his own anymore in their home. He feels fortunate to have found a reliable, pleasant housekeeper, but is very weary of the continuing burden of his wife's care.

Although he has witnessed his wife's loss of memory, Mr. Barnett has not trained himself to give up old patterns of communication. For example, upon coming home in the evening he will say, just to make conversation, "What did you have for lunch today?" Then he is upset once again by his wife's inability to remember. Simply put, he has not accomplished the basic task of accepting what he cannot change.

Mr. Barnett feels sorry for his wife, who is very docile and very affectionate with him, but no longer able to be a companion or to take part in conversation. He is torn apart by the mindless chatter of his once witty, intelligent partner. He is even sorrier for himself.

Discussion

Is this the best solution for Mr. and Mrs. Barnett? What else can be done?

In the early stage of Mrs. Barnett's illness, her husband did not recognize the serious memory loss she suffered and the extent of the resulting confusion. When he left written instructions to peel the potatoes or wash the salad at a particular time, it seemed like a simple way to keep his wife occupied. Instead, it led to increased frustration and agitated behavior.

Imagine for an instant the feelings of someone who reads "Peel the potatoes at 4 o'clock and put them in a pot of water" if she no longer knows what time it is or where the potatoes are kept, or perhaps what potatoes are; if she doesn't remember what the word *peel* means or where the pots are, and how to put water in one. It is a complicated scenario for a severely forgetful, confused older person, and can understandably lead to upset, excited behavior.

In Mrs. Barnett's case, the disturbed behavior could have been anticipated. Luckily, Mr. Barnett did not let more than one month go by with excessive telephone bills until he learned how to control the situation. He was fortunate in getting her to a medical evaluation, which led to a prescription for medication that made her behavior more manageable. Remember, however, that this was not done as part of a plan to help him care for her at home. It came about by chance, as part of the application process for nursing-home care. His children, while telling him vehemently that he must not put her in a nursing home, were not able to help with advice to take her to a doctor who might medicate her, since they were not knowledgeable in this area. Most people are not. But this actually turned out to be the best course of action at that time.

Mr. Barnett now understands and accepts his wife's behavior, since he has made every effort to learn about the nature of her condition. But even though he has learned to accept it, he is still very upset by the whole situation. He feels he would be much better off if she were in a nursing home, but he recognizes that even if cost were not a factor, he might not be able to go through with a placement opposed by his children. He feels resentful and defeated.

Mr. Barnett's children have been so upset by their mother's mental changes and their own personal problems that they have failed to recognize what is happening to their father. He might benefit if they would encourage him to take an extended vacation, perhaps to a health resort or spa where he can work on his own health problems. If the children do not assume a protective role in relation to their father at this time, they may find that he will not survive this stressful state for long.

Since Mr. Barnett's experience with exploring the possibility of a nursing home placement, regulations about Medicaid eligibility and the financial responsibility of spouses have changed. Although many nursing homes do not inform applicants about it, when someone enters an institution for long-term care, only the income and assets that are in the name of the resident/patient have to be used for their care. Income and assets belonging to the non-institutionalized spouse do not have to be turned over to the nursing home.

These regulations are not even known to many professionals working in the field of aging, so it is important for family members to make themselves knowledgeable about this. Be sure to consult a Medicaid office for the most recent regulations concerning your entitlements.

MR. AND MRS. GOLD

Mr. Gold is an eighty-one-year-old, Russian-born retired printer from Canada. He and his wife moved to a mobile-home community in Florida sixteen years ago, after his retirement. They were married twenty-three years ago, after both were widowed. Mrs. Gold is an intelligent, charming, eighty-one-year-old French Canadian whose only son is a professor living in Montreal. Mr. Gold had a son and daughter from his first marriage, who both live in Toronto.

Mr. and Mrs. Gold were very happy together. They

each had modest savings, and pooling their resources made it possible to purchase their mobile home and enjoy the pleasant climate in Florida. They were active in their community and church, enjoying relatively good health until four years ago, when Mrs. Gold fell and fractured her hip. Since then she has walked very slowly, and only for short distances. She looks very fragile and weighs less than ninety-five pounds. At the same time that Mrs. Gold was recovering from her fracture and was dependent upon her husband to assist her, she became aware that his memory, which had been failing, was becoming worse. At times he seemed quite confused.

Over the next two years Mr. Gold's mental condition deteriorated, and even his personality seemed to change. He had previously been an "old world gentleman," courtly, intelligent, interested in world politics and literary discussions. As his memory deteriorated, he was no longer able to read a book or even to follow the news on television. At times sweet and loving, he became increasingly irritable and argumentative.

The doctor told Mrs. Gold that her husband was suffering from "hardening of the arteries," and gave him some medication to improve his circulation. Mrs. Gold makes sure he takes his medication, including something for diabetes, which he has been taking for years. Gradually, Mrs. Gold had to take over supervising her husband's bathing and dressing as he became unable to perform the most routine functions.

Mrs. Gold has been finding the extra work burdensome, and her son, who is devoted to her, has suggested that she come to live with him and his wife and let Mr. Gold's children take care of him. She didn't want to abandon her husband, but she did go to her son's for a month's vacation to regain her strength. Mr. Gold's daughter took him to her home during that period, but he was very disoriented, and it was so difficult to take care of him that Mr. Gold's children called Mrs. Gold at her son's home several times, pleading with her to cut short the vacation so that they could bring their father home. But her son insisted that she stay until she was stronger.

When Mrs. Gold went back home and Mr. Gold's son brought him back, the son offered to send fifty dollars a week so that she could hire someone to help with the house. He has been sending this amount for the past two years, which has been a help, but Mr. Gold has gotten much worse in the interim.

Mr. Gold doesn't dare go out of the house, since he is aware of his confusion. Sometimes he lapses into his native Russian, which Mrs. Gold doesn't understand, and at times he seems unable to understand English or French, in which he had been fluent.

Mr. Gold was always well groomed and proper. Now he sometimes refuses to shave. He claimed at one point that his electric shaver was faulty, so Mrs. Gold bought him a new one. Still he would refuse to shave for days at a time and would curse and use offensive language she had never heard him use before in response to her questions about his appearance.

He has also developed some habits that his wife finds disgusting, such as spitting on the floor. They have carpeting on the floor, and even the housekeeper who comes in once a week cannot clean up such a mess. Mrs. Gold cannot understand why he cannot remember to use a tissue if he must spit. She is also upset because he cannot remember to lift the toilet seat when he urinates, and she finds herself screaming at him when she must clean up after him. When Mr. Gold coughs or sneezes, he never remembers to use his handkerchief.

At times Mr. Gold is aware of the trouble he is causing his wife, and he is very sorry. Once she left him to bathe, and when he came out of the bathtub he told her that he was thinking that he should drown himself because he really loved her. Mrs. Gold reassured him that she loved him too and certainly didn't want him to drown himself. Still, she wonders how long she can go on like this.

One aspect of caring for Mr. Gold that is particularly upsetting and puzzling is that he has become very distrustful of her at times. When she withdraws money from their joint bank account to pay for their rent or other expenses, he accuses her of using up all their savings. When she tries to explain where the money is going, he becomes enraged and says she is stealing it for herself.

When he had to sign a lease renewal recently, he refused, even though she pointed out that they would be evicted otherwise. She explained the problem to the manager of their mobile home community, and when he came and told Mr. Gold that he would have to sign or move out, Mr. Gold meekly signed. This made Mrs. Gold feel that her husband can behave reasonably with others and is only angry with her for some unknown reason.

Another particularly troubling problem for Mrs. Gold is that every meal has become a source of stress. Mr. Gold complains that all the food tastes terrible, even when they go out to eat. At breakfast he tries to use ten or twelve packages of artificial sweetener on his cereal. Every day Mrs. Gold argues with him that two packages are enough and that he'll get sick if he uses such an abnormal amount of sweetener, but Mr. Gold becomes very angry with her, telling her that she can't tell him what to do. Sometimes, in retaliation, he refuses to eat at all. Mrs. Gold realizes that something's wrong with her husband, but she cannot really accept the fact that he cannot change his behavior, and so the same upsetting scene is repeated seven days a week. She and her husband eat less and less, and both are losing considerable weight.

Mrs. Gold does not want to give up her home and enter an institution with her husband, as was suggested when she turned to a family counseling agency for some extra assistance at home. Mrs. Gold does not want to put her husband in a nursing home, since this would make her feel too guilty. Since their income is slightly above the level of eligibility for Medicaid, the family counseling agency said they could not secure home help except on a private basis. Mrs. Gold is afraid to spend any more of their income for help.

Discussion

Although Mr. and Mrs. Gold visit their doctor regularly, he has not taken the time to listen to all the problems she has described to him. He has not explained, for instance, that even Mr. Gold's complaints about food might be a result of changes in his brain function. They can also be related to changes in his taste buds. The combination of physical changes in his taste buds, which are part of the aging process, and mental changes, which make it impossible for him to understand the physical changes, leads to his difficult behavior at mealtime.

A brief explanation from the physician, which is not any more than good medical practice, could clarify the nature of the mealtime problem. A concerned physician would elicit information that would reveal Mr. Gold's

paranoid behavior toward his wife, which might be relieved by the appropriate tranquilizer. In addition, he
should make a referral to a visiting nurse for a home management assessment, which might ease many of the problems for a while.

The person responsible for feeding a mentally impaired older person must learn to anticipate the problems
we have described, and to simplify the rituals of mealtime.
Salt, pepper, sugar, sweeteners, mustard, ketchup, relish,
and so on should be kept out of sight. Only one item of
food should be put out at one time, since the impaired
person often has forgotten the usual order of eating. For
example, if a tray is made up with soup, salad, main
course, and dessert, the impaired person often eats the
dessert first and may not have any appetite for the rest of
the meal.

It may take a great deal of experimenting to find foods
that please the mentally impaired older person whose
sense of taste is also impaired. Mr. Gold's needs are further complicated by his diabetes. Mrs. Gold might try to
flavor his cereal with cinnamon or other spices, or mix it
with artificially sweetened jellies. Sometimes an entirely
different type of flavor might work; she might, for instance, add sugar-free chocolate to the cereal. The best
solution of all might be to switch from cereal altogether in
the morning and offer something different, such as a sand-
wich. Mrs. Gold could use counseling and guidance in the
changing nutritional needs and challenges she will face in
feeding her mentally impaired spouse. Public health
nurses are very good at providing this type of counseling,
but not enough people know about the services of such
outstanding agencies as the Visiting Nurse Service.

Appendix 1 contains lists of management principles

for supervising and providing for the safety, health, and nutritional needs of your mentally impaired relative at home. These charts can serve as a guide for Mrs. Gold and others struggling with similar problems. But they will not eliminate her emotional response to her husband's erratic behavior.

Because she and her husband are so obviously failing, they clearly need more help in order to prevent some serious illness or accident. They need help at least three times a week to support their present level of functioning, and at present Mrs. Gold has help only once a week.

When an older couple experiences such decline, there is often confusion and conflict among their children as to who in the family should do what and for how long. Old resentments and rivalries may surface as the family struggles with the crisis. In the case of a crisis for a couple in a second marriage, especially where there are children of both former marriages, the confusion and resentments may be even more complicated. (Not necessarily, of course. Some step-families are as caring and responsible as natural families.)

What we usually see in such cases is the expectation that the children feel responsible primarily for their own parent. This is often a source of conflict and should be talked out openly, in the interest of arriving at the best possible plan for the parents. The capacities of both sets of children must be considered, as well as the degree of burden presented by the impaired parent.

In addition, to help cope with the emotional trauma she experiences daily, Mrs. Gold could benefit from having someone with whom she could talk out her feelings. The family is geographically distant. There are too few professional counselors available who might be able to help Mrs. Gold deal with her feelings on a continuing basis. Neighbors are usually unable to help someone with this type of long-term problem because they often feel helpless in the face of such tragedy and try to avoid talking about it, or offer inappropriate advice if they have not experienced a similar problem.

A very effective source of help would be a support group in Mrs. Gold's local community—a group of people with similar problems who meet in an area that is accessible to her. Talking out her despair about the changes in her husband's condition with others who can understand and share her pain would ease the pain and strengthen her ability to cope. Such groups exist, however, in not as many cities as needed, having just begun a few years ago. Chapter 12 will describe how such groups work, with practical suggestions for how to locate them or how to start them in communities where they are needed.

MR. MARSHALL

Mr. Marshall, a seventy-three-year-old retired business-man, was diagnosed about three years ago as suffering from Alzheimer's disease. At that time he gave up going to his office and turned the business over to his son. He lives in a comfortable house in a large Midwestern city, where he is well known as a civic and community leader. His sixty-year-old wife and his thirty-year-old daughter live with him. His married son visits once a week.

Mr. Marshall was always known for his quick wit and original sense of humor, but since he's become aware of his loss of memory and occasional confusion, he has become glum and nervous. He smokes constantly. Mrs. Marshall is irritable and short-tempered with him, responding sharply to his repetitious questions. She is even more upset by her own behavior than by her husband's, because she knows he can't change his, and she feels she should be able to control hers. Her husband seems sorrowful when she blows up at him, but in seconds he has forgotten the incident and continues with his repetitious, anxious questioning. Their daughter works all day and has a busy social life, so she is not much help to Mrs. Marshall. Their son is preoccupied with running the family business and makes his weekly visits as short as possible.

One serious source of anxiety for the family is the danger posed by Mr. Marshall's smoking. Once, when Mr. Marshall dozed off in front of the TV set, his cigarette fell out of his hand and set fire to the carpet. Luckily, Mrs. Marshall smelled the smoke before any serious damage was done, but the incident made her aware of the possibility of more hazardous consequences. She has tried to keep cigarettes away from Mr. Marshall since then, but nothing works.

Mrs. Marshall is also in constant fear that he will have an automobile accident, but she is unable to tell him to give up driving because she feels this will strip him of his last sense of masculinity and control. Other members of the family are very upset about this situation, because sometimes Mr. Marshall drives with his small grandchildren in the car. Their daughter-in-law has said that she will no longer allow the children to ride with him.

Discussion

Which problems require immediate solutions? How can the Marshalls behave more responsibly?

This case is an example of how the family can sometimes be so emotionally disturbed by this devastating illness that they are unable to take the commonsense steps necessary to ensure basic safety. Any outsider looking at this situation can see that if Mr. Marshall's memory and judgment are now so impaired that it is unsafe for his grandchildren to ride with him, it is also unsafe for anyone else to ride with him or to be on the road or in the street while he is driving. Yet no one in the family had the courage to confront him. They were so overwhelmed with grief over what had become of this successful head of the household that they were incapable of rational behavior. They were unable to assume the responsible role demanded by the changes in Mr. Marshall in order to protect him and the rest of his family and community.

This problem can be handled rationally, but first the family must get beyond its emotional roadblocks.

A first step toward management of this problem is a consultation with the physician for a professional confirmation that it's no longer safe for the impaired older person to drive. If the physician recommends that Mr. Marshall stop driving, the family will have less of a feeling of personally hurting him, and can accomplish the task in a more matter-of-fact manner. The family must make arrangements for others to drive Mr. Marshall around. (This practical necessity often leads a family to put off taking action, delaying sometimes until a catastrophe takes place.)

If the mentally impaired older person is uncooperative about giving up driving, it is up to the family to make sure that he cannot drive. A mechanic will demonstrate how to remove parts of the car easily so that it cannot be driven. Removing the distributor cap, for example, may solve the problem. If the impaired older person becomes frustrated and disruptive, the family must be prepared for special handling. Very often the person can be distracted by an alternative task or event, such as mowing the lawn together, or sitting down for a cup of coffee. The issue of the car will then be forgotten. One family I knew had a prepared box of simple crafts that was always successful in distracting their father when he was frustrated and otherwise unreachable.

The issue of Mr. Marshall's smoking requires family action as well. It is essential that smoking be permitted only when he can be supervised. Many modern fabrics can be instantly set afire, and an old person with lowered recuperative powers might not survive being injured badly by a burning acrylic shirt, for example. It is urgent that impaired smokers be closely monitored for their own safety and for the peace of mind of their families. Monitoring involves a responsible person keeping the cigarettes of the smoker and doling them out only when someone is available to supervise. This is a very difficult task for some family members who emotionally view this as another assault on the independence of their loved one. In a society that stresses the democratic values of freedom and independence, it is very difficult to take away these rights of adult relatives. The family member confronted with such a task must focus on the *purpose* of the monitoring, which is the safety of his loved one and others.

The most practical thing would be to try to get the impaired older person to give up smoking. Although difficult at first, it might make the most sense to prohibit cigarettes altogether. The physician might, for instance, prescribe some tranquilizer to get the smoker through the withdrawal period. At the same time, family members should use ingenuity in coming up with some substitute activity, such as increased exercise, listening to favorite old records, or working on simple craft projects. Mrs. Marshall might enlist her daughter and son to take her husband for long walks or to create a project that would occupy him for a while. The primary care-giver in a family must learn how to ask other available members to share responsibility, with suggestions as to how they can contribute their special skills in developing a family care plan.

MRS. JAMES

Mrs. James is a seventy-nine-year-old woman who was deserted by her husband forty years ago. Her five living children range in age from fifty-nine to forty-five. Four live in New York, and all are employed full time. She lives in a house in New Jersey with her youngest daughter, Ann, who is a nurse, divorced. Ann's children are away at college. While her grandchildren were growing up, Mrs. James did most of the cooking, cleaning, and baby-sitting. After they left, she had very little to occupy her. She became very confused over a period of about a year, constantly rummaging through the house, going through drawers and misplacing things. Her daughter often couldn't find her watch, her jewelry, her comfortable shoes, but her mother denied even touching them. Sometimes, when Ann took a cup from the cupboard, she would find her mother's dentures in it.

The family, which is close-knit, tried to share the burden, taking turns having Mrs. James visit, but as soon as she arrived in the home of one of her other children, Mrs. James would say she wanted to go home and refuse to unpack her suitcase. Back home with Ann, she would start her rummaging again.

Mrs. James's confusion has caused considerable trouble. One day Ann came home to find she couldn't get into the house. The key wouldn't open the door. It turned out that when Mrs. James came back from a walk, she wasn't able to open the door—she was using the wrong key—so she let herself in through the garage, which was open, and called a locksmith to change the lock on the front door.

Another time, Ann came home to find all her favorite sweaters and dresses missing. Mrs. James had packed them up and mailed them to some nieces in Chicago. Apparently she sent them to the wrong address, since they never came back.

The family hired a companion to keep her out of trouble, but Mrs. James sent her away, saying that she didn't need a baby-sitter. At times she is quite alert and assertive about what she wants. Her children have tried to persuade her to go into a nursing home, where she would not be alone all day, but Mrs. James assures them that she took care of all of them and her grandchildren, and she can certainly take care of herself.

Discussion

What did Mrs. James's family do that added to her confusion? What other solutions might they seek?

When Mrs. James refused to stay at the home of her other children, she was not just being stubborn or showing favoritism. She just wanted to be in familiar surroundings. As an older person's memory fails, it is important for him to maintain familiar routines. A moderately impaired older person may manage for quite a long time if established routines can be followed. Mrs. James realized instinctively that she was more confused in the homes of her other children and therefore under more stress. Although their intentions were good in trying to share the burden of their sister Ann, moving from place to place was too much of a disruption for their mother, whose fragile mental state made her totally dependent on the known cues in her own home and neighborhood.

Mrs. James's behavior at home certainly indicates that she needs supervision and some routinized activities to occupy her during the day. One possible solution might be to find a day-care center that offers a specialized program for impaired older persons. If the program is individually designed to involve the mentally impaired client, and the staff is skillful in helping the resistant older person to ad-just, such a setting might work for Mrs. James, at least for a while. Unfortunately, since there are so few programs available at this time that meet these criteria, such a solu-tion is more hypothetical than practical.

The few day-care programs that currently exist are pri-marily for the physically impaired and are based on a med-ical model, which makes them costly. The even fewer that serve the mentally impaired are so limited they can usually offer service for only two or three days a week. This is not sufficient for the older person whose relatives work and who is otherwise alone, or whose relatives are worn out by the burden of twenty-four-hour care. There is an urgent need for day-care centers with programs geared to the capacities of the mentally impaired aged. As relatives of the mentally impaired aged in the community meet one another through other support groups, they may find it productive to organize demand for day-care programs. They must search out what is available in their own com-munities, and then make their needs known to the powers that be. An innovative group of relatives can start their own program, and show the professionals what needs to be done. (See chapter 12.)

Mrs. James's family faces the same dilemmas as Mrs. Wells's family—though at an earlier stage—even though Mrs. Wells lives alone and Mrs. James lives with a daughter. Her mental impairment is clearly getting steadily worse. Most of the time she is alone and at constant risk of doing something harmful to herself or to others. She has demonstrated her forgetfulness, confusion, and faulty judgment. Even though she usually seems to be functioning normally, it takes only one mistake to cause a hazardous situation. For example, were she to go out in winter without adequate clothing and then become confused about her whereabouts, wandering for hours, she would probably end up with pneumonia.

It does not make sense simply to wait for a catastrophe, although it is very tempting to a family who feels its efforts are unappreciated. The family must overcome its sense of helplessness and keep trying to provide the care required. If the first few attempts at home help are rejected or sabotaged, perhaps the next ones won't be. Ask yourself this: Whose persistence can last longer—a united family, determined to provide care, or an obstinate, independent old person who no longer knows what is good for him? Whatever the outcome, the responsible family must know that they are doing their best. If unsuccessful at present, they must plan a tentative strategy for the future, knowing that nothing stays the same—the only certain thing is change.

MRS. COOPER

Mrs. Cooper is an eighty-three-year-old widow who has lived in Arizona for the past fifteen years, in a private house next door to her widowed sister. Her sister died six months ago, and since then Mrs. Cooper's only daughter, Jane, who lives on the West Coast, has become concerned about her ability to function alone. Jane was aware that her mother's memory was slipping, but as long as the sister lived next door, there was no problem. Recently the housekeeper called to say that Mrs. Cooper had been served a subpoena to appear in court for nonpayment of bills. It turned out that Mrs. Cooper had been ordering things from a department store, running up a very large bill, and then not responding to their monthly reminders. They finally closed her charge account and were taking her to court.

When Jane discussed this with her mother, Mrs. Cooper seemed unaware of the whole situation. Eventually Jane found out that her mother's sister had been managing Mrs. Cooper's finances for several years, occasionally returning things to the department store when Mrs. Cooper would order the same things twice. Jane's aunt had been protecting her from the knowledge that her mother had become mentally incompetent and totally dependent on her sister. With the sister's sudden death, Mrs. Cooper's problems surfaced.

As Jane investigated her mother's financial situation, she discovered that her mother's taxes were unpaid and that her utilities were about to be turned off. Fortunately the housekeeper was an honest, reliable woman who had helped Mrs. Cooper by cashing her social security and annuity checks, which took care of the regular expenses of running the house. However, Jane found a pile of unopened letters, including dividend checks.

Jane felt uncomfortable about suggesting to her mother that they go to the bank together so that the accounts could be put in both names. She was not interested in her mother's money and told her so. But she was practical enough to realize that she had to assume responsibility for her mother's financial affairs, since she couldn't afford to pay a lawyer to handle them. Her mother was grateful to her daughter for coming to her rescue. At the bank, an officer suggested that Mrs. Cooper give her daughter power of attorney so that she could handle other business matters for her mother if necessary. This was arranged at the bank.

Jane was able to determine from the housekeeper and from her mother's neighbors that there didn't seem to be any other problems. Mrs. Cooper visited regularly with her neighbors, who were sympathetic and helpful. Her health was good and she took no medications. She expressed a preference for staying in her own home with her pet cats rather than being uprooted by moving closer to her daughter, but she agreed to have all her mail delivered to her daughter's address so that she could take care of her affairs more easily. Jane was able to return home with the sense that everything was under control for the time being.

Discussion

Was there anything else Jane should have done? Since Mrs. Cooper had a reliable housekeeper and good neighbors, her basic needs were met. Jane could allow her mother to continue living in her own home, since this was her preference. This situation was comparatively simple because Mrs. Cooper's confusion was primarily in the area of finances and the problem was discovered before a devastating amount of financial losses occurred.

Families must be aware of this particularly vulnerable area, because there are strong feelings that sometimes keep relatives from taking charge of finances. Many people are afraid that in taking control of finances they may be accused of trying to get their relative's money. This can become absurd when family members see funds misused, lost, or squandered, and are embarrassed to take action for fear that their motives will be misinterpreted. This is foolish and irresponsible behavior, yet it occurs often.

It is important that families contact an attorney while their relative is still competent to sign a "durable power of attorney," which enables the designated responsible person to manage their finances should the need arise. If your relative is unable to accept this practicality, you may have to engage an attorney to apply to the courts to determine and initiate the required protective actions. (See the section on legal services in Appendix 3.)

Even when the impaired older person has limited funds, the family may have to take financial responsibility. If the person has only social security and is incapable of managing these funds, a responsible relative can apply to social security to become the payee of the funds, guaranteeing to spend these on behalf of the older person. By anticipating this as a problem area, the responsible relative can avoid such traumas as eviction notices, telephone service interruptions, and cutoffs of gas, electricity, and fuel delivery.

These six case examples are composites of real people dealing with real problems. They have been selected as typical of many of the challenges that face the readers of this book. The basic principles for caring for your relative at home are summarized in Appendix 1, but it would be impossible, of course, to identify all of the variations of possible problems that might confront you as your relative continues to decline. Who could predict, for example, the behavior of one lady who cut off the stems of all her daughter's plants and put them in the freezer so that they would last longer? Or the gentleman who stopped eating anything but potatoes, explaining that "they have such cute eyes." Or the countless ways false teeth and eyeglasses can be misplaced?

What you must learn, therefore, is to be prepared for anything. Try to laugh as much as possible at some of the bizarre behavior. This is not laughing at someone who can't help himself, but at a situation that is ludicrous. Humor is one of the most effective therapeutic outlets, but it's not easy to smile when you're exhausted. When all else fails, perhaps you can laugh at yourself for trying to be perfect.

In much of this chapter, you may have noticed similarities to behavioral problems in child psychology. References to handling children have been avoided, even though some of the techniques discussed in Appendix 2 are based upon the same principles. However, in child care you are dealing with developmental tasks. With education, love, and discipline, the child can be taught how to behave socially. He will learn and grow. The impaired older person is the opposite of a child, even though his behavior is sometimes similar. He cannot learn as the child does, because his brain function is impaired. He will not mature and grow. He will deteriorate. This tragic irony explains in part your conflicting emotions as you try to find new ways to relate to your kin.

7

Paranoia

*I*t is very difficult to relate to someone who is no longer normal. We have many explicit rules of conduct, and when someone in the street starts shouting at some unseen enemy, we try to get as far away as possible.

These same feelings are called forth when the older person you are concerned about loses touch with reality, displaying a pattern of disordered thinking. When you realize that your rational explanations do not penetrate the new reality your kin has adopted, it makes you want to get as far away as possible.

For example, Mrs. Arnold became convinced that the superintendent of the apartment house where she had lived for over thirty years was directing some electrical impulses through the radiators in her apartment. She said that the electricity was causing a buzzing in her head and making her dizzy and nauseated. She complained about this by telephone to her daughter at work, at least twice a day. The daughter, recognizing this as an abnormal mental process, tried to reassure her mother. She said that they had known the superintendent for many years, and he had always been helpful and friendly. The more she tried to persuade her mother that she was mistaken, the more insistent her mother became that the superintendent was the source of all her problems. She grew so agitated that she became abusive to the superintendent, ringing his doorbell at all hours, screaming at him in the halls in front of other tenants and threatening to report him to the landlord. She even called the police, who advised the daughter to get Mrs. Arnold to a doctor before she was evicted. Mrs. Arnold refused to go to a doctor, screaming, "I'm not crazy. Just lock up the super so he won't make me sick anymore."

Mrs. Arnold seemed perfectly rational except for this fixation. That made it all the harder for her daughter to deal with.

Sometimes an older person starts to experience a physical change, usually a decline in some faculty, which he does not recognize as such—a buzzing in the head, for example, or hearing loss, or difficulty in moving about. Some people seem to need to blame others for such changes, being unable to accept the possibility that some failure within themselves is responsible. This need to blame others is a primitive psychological defense; it's used early in life as an excuse for personal failure, until we learn to accept responsibility for our own actions as part of the process of growing up. But if we are too demanding of ourselves, or if greater demands are made of us than we can achieve, we may still occasionally rationalize our failures away by blaming others, sometimes at an unconscious level, sometimes openly.

Even when we are unaware of this psychological process, however, it is usually bound by the limits of realistic possibilities. For instance, a normal, rational person knows that buzzing sounds in the head are not caused by electrical impulses being sent through the radiators. When someone in old age adopts such an irrational explanation for physical changes, we might infer that the part of the brain that makes judgments and sorts fact from fiction is malfunctioning. Therefore, no amount of rational explanation or clarification makes sense to the impaired older person. This unrealistic blaming behavior is what we call a paranoid reaction.

Trying to persuade a disturbed older person that the person he is convinced is trying to destroy him is really harmless is one of the most frustrating processes imaginable. The older person's response is usually the firm conviction that he is right, and the relative who is trying to be protective and understanding often ends up feeling rejected, mistrusted, abused.

If this is one of your problems, what should you do? As a first step, you must understand that the older person who fastens upon a bizarre explanation for events is trying to make some sense out of what appear to him to be confusing and frightening changes. The more you try to strip away the irrational explanation, the more frightened and anxious he will become. It is very important to recognize the *anxiety* behind the behavior.

This behavior seems to occur more frequently in people who experience sensory losses, particularly hearing problems, although no one knows why. One possible explanation is that an older person who becomes hard of hearing is often embarrassed and tries to conceal it. He may mis-hear what is being said to him, or to others, and may misinterpret or distort what is being said. This distorted perception of what he has heard may develop into a belief that something negative is being said to or about him.

In my own geriatric practice I experienced a vivid example of how a hearing problem can relate to paranoid behavior. A suspicious, hostile resident in a senior housing project was referred to a psychiatrist because of problems she was creating. She had refused to pay her rent for some months because of alleged mistreatment, and she had alienated all the other residents with her dour expression and sarcastic remarks. At times she became agitated to the point of threatening the other residents with a cane. At the end of a session with the psychiatrist, who had managed to talk with her in spite of her severe hearing problem, she was told, "You're very nervous, and I'm going to give you some medicine to calm you down. You're to take it three times a day. It's called Thorazine." The resident misheard the name Thorazine for "poison" and ran through the halls screaming, "Poison! Poison! I won't take it!"

Nothing could convince her that the doctor did not plan to poison her, but in time she responded to a social worker who demonstrated her understanding of the resident's fears and offered to protect her.

TYPICAL PARANOID REACTIONS

Paranoid behavior can take many forms, but there do seem to be several common types.

Money Matters

One of the most frequent sources of paranoid ideas in old age is suspiciousness about money. This occurs with people who have lots of money, people who no longer have as much money as they once had, and people who have never had any great amount of money. Since money represents power and independence, it can be a significant issue all through our lives, but in old age it frequently is a source of anxiety, particularly when the older person's mental faculties are failing.

One of the tasks of the family is to become protective as its elderly member becomes impaired. When the older person's memory and judgment fail, and he has money and other assets in his name, the family has the responsibility to take steps in protecting the assets. Very often, family members delay taking sensible steps in this direction for fear that they will be accused of being interested in their relative's money. (See chapter 10 for the discussion of assuming responsibility for finances or for arranging for protection of assets.)

A Protestant minister once came to see me about a problem concerning his aged father. The father, who lived in a separate apartment house, took his meals with the minister and his wife, but otherwise he maintained his independence, employing a housekeeper to clean his apartment and do his laundry. As it became apparent that the old man had grown very forgetful and sometimes confused, the minister suggested that his father put his bank account in both their names so that he could pay his bills for him. The father developed the idea that his son was planning to cheat him and refused. Every time a check had to be signed for the rent or the housekeeper, the father claimed that his son was tricking him. At times the father became enraged and threatened to call in the FBI. The minister was so upset by his father's accusations that he sometimes paid the bills himself. This upset his wife, since he really couldn't afford to pay the additional bills on his modest salary.

Although he recognized that the changes in his father's behavior were related to his advanced years (he was over ninety), the minister's eyes filled with tears as he told me that he couldn't understand how his father's mind could become so twisted as to mistrust his only son, a man of religion, a man who had the faith and confidence of all his parishioners. The minister was so hurt by his father's suspicions that he had become hopelessly frustrated by his problem, not knowing what to do next.

Further discussion revealed that his father, a very learned professor from a well-to-do background, had always been the stern head of the family. He was accustomed to being treated with deference, first for his professional status and family position, and then for his advanced age. He had raised his son to be frugal and independent, and he was always secretive about his plans for the family fortune. Although his mental impairment was apparent to others, he could not accept these changes in himself, and so, to fill in the gaps about his financial situation caused by his faulty memory, he developed the idea that his son was trying to trick him, to retaliate for his lack of generosity with the family money.

Because of his emotional involvement, the minister could not recognize that he had resented his father's attitude for most of his life and was tormented by guilt for the depth of his anger. Instead, he stated that he admired and loved his father and was grateful for his disciplined upbringing. This inability to understand his complex feelings in relation to his father—the anger along with the admiration, and a chronic problem with guilt—led to his inability to take appropriate steps to safeguard his father's money.

Although the minister did not have the emotional energy to work through his lifelong problem with his father, with counseling he was able to identify those parts of the problem that he could handle during the current crisis. He came to see that his father's behavior was not simply a normal consequence of old age, but rather that it was related to an illness that might respond to medical treatment. The daughter-in-law was able to persuade him to see his doctor on the basis of his poor color and unsteadiness. It turned out that he had become anemic, which of course meant a decrease in the amount of oxygen available to the brain. With treatment, his behavior improved somewhat, although his memory didn't. The doctor prescribed a tranquilizer, which made him more amenable to the son's suggestion that an officer of the bank take responsibility for paying his bills every month. Although the family situation was not ideal, it had become more manageable.

It is very important for families to recognize that a realistic concern about money, from worries about the cost of care to the preservation of assets, is a normal consideration. It should not be denied because of the uncomfortable feelings that money usually provokes. These are natural feelings, and they can be put in proper perspective if we recognize them. This principle can be particularly helpful when trying to sort out your emotions concerning your elderly relative who, as you try to help, may become suspicious of your motives.

Lost and Found

An older person whose memory is failing usually misplaces things—keys, eyeglasses, sweaters. Often, things that are of most value are put away in a "safe place" so they won't get lost. When the memory loss is very severe, the older person might not recall that he had even handled any of these items. And if his tendency is to be suspicious, he might conclude that the items were stolen, usually focusing on someone in particular. Again, you can see how the relationship of some physiological loss (memory impairment), a personality characteristic (suspiciousness), and impaired judgment could lead to a mistaken perception of reality.

Try to avoid confronting your relative with the obviousness of the false accusation that the neighbor is stealing his eyeglasses. "What would Mrs. Green do with your eyeglasses?" would probably cause your relative to be upset in an instant. It would be better to ignore comments about the neighbor and say, "It must feel terrible to be without your eyeglasses. Let's keep searching together to see if we can find them." When the missing item is found, don't try to teach your relative a lesson by saying, "See, they were only mislaid. Now you can see that Mrs. Green didn't steal them." Your relative will not be able to understand the lesson. Just reinforce the positive feeling attached to finding the missing eyeglasses by saying something like "Now we both feel better."

Sometimes you will find yourself saying something to your relative that you know will upset him, even as you say it. Although wanting intellectually to reassure him of your concern, you may express anger instead. You may hear yourself complaining, "Why are you so quick to accuse someone of taking your things when you know you're always misplacing everything?" Knowing that your relative can't change his behavior will make you feel guilty about your response. However, if you recognize that it was the only response you were able to come up with at the time and that it was a way of releasing your upset feelings over your kin's decline, you should be magnanimous enough to forgive yourself! Besides, your relative's likely response would be to refute your comment by saying, "It *was* stolen. But he put it back when we weren't looking because he knew you had come to help me."

The key to understanding paranoid ideas is to see them as a reaction to a confusing and distorted environment. Such reactions serve a purpose for your impaired kin. If you can laugh to yourself, or with others, over the fanciful ideas your relative comes up with, it would help enormously.

The staff of an excellent nursing home was very upset over the incidence of several cases of scabies on the floor that housed the most confused patients. This called for a complete scouring of that whole section of the institution. Every patient had to be bathed with a special antiseptic, every item of clothing had to be removed and sterilized, and all the bed linens, drapes, pillows, and mattresses had to be cleaned and sterilized. The harassed staff had explained the procedure and the reason for it to all the patients and relatives, but because of the patients' state of confusion and forgetfulness, they could not understand the turmoil taking place. In the midst of all the work, one ancient patient who returned from his bath to find his room bare came padding down the corridor in his disposable slippers, hospital gown flapping behind him. He pounded on the desk of the nurses' station. "I want someone to call the police," he shouted. "I'm here to report the most colossal case of thievery I have ever experienced in my entire life."

The staff found it a lot easier to cope with the rest of the day when they could laugh together over the patient's interpretation of the results of their hard work.

Hallucinations and Delusions

When a mentally impaired older person's senses fail, he may see or hear things that are not there, but that are real to him, nevertheless. Sometimes an old person who is somewhat isolated hears voices that he is convinced are real, even though there is no person attached to the voices. If the old person is suffering from depressive feelings, the voices might add to his feelings of worthlessness or to his anxiety. Sometimes a disturbed older person hears voices that accuse him of terrible deeds, or tell him he is dirty, or that he has a horrible disease. On the other hand, the voices may be reassuring and grand—discussions with angels or other larger-than-life beings that offer protection or suggestions for actions.

Mrs. Bennet, a native New Yorker, complained bitterly to her daughter that the Hungarians had gotten into her television set and were speaking Hungarian on her favorite channel. "They're having a big parade with gypsies," she insisted, "and now they'll ruin the neighborhood." When her daughter protested, Mrs. Bennet was very matter-of-fact in stating, "Well, turn on the channel and you'll see for yourself."

What should the daughter's response be? Again, confrontation is wrong. Understanding and reassurance can be given without agreeing with what her mother is seeing and hearing. "I can understand that must be very annoying to you even though I don't hear it" would probably meet the mother's immediate need. Then the daughter should be sure that Mrs. Bennet's doctor is told that she's hallucinating. The doctor would probably check on whether anything could help her vision or hearing and whether any medication she was taking might produce this symptom as a side effect. He might then prescribe something to relieve the symptom as well as the distress caused by the symptom.

Sometimes the best response is no response. Mrs. Korn told her children that her husband was lying on the living room couch all day and all night. She said she talked to him but he wouldn't answer because he was very tired. Since her husband had been dead for several years, this news really upset them. Mrs. Korn, however, was apparently not upset by this experience, discussing it very casually, and in time it disappeared without treatment.

Some impaired old people develop jealous delusions, a kind of second cousin to a persecution complex. With no apparent basis in fact, the old person can become fixated on the idea that the relative who cares for him doesn't pay enough attention to him or doesn't love him enough. If the relative even talks to someone else, the old person can erupt into a jealous rage. This delusion does not often respond to reassurances. Again, the jealous obsession must be understood as a symptom of some underlying anxiety, and the old person should be treated medically if at all possible.

Sometimes the older person whose sense of smell or taste has changed becomes convinced that something is being done to his food or that certain gases are being released to harm him. He may insist that someone is trying to poison him, and he may become so fearful that he refuses to eat at all. Obviously this behavior requires immediate treatment. If nothing else can calm his fears, hospitalization may be necessary.

Occasionally the older person who is afraid he's being poisoned might try to protect himself by hurting the one who he thinks is harming him. It is important not to panic in the face of this behavior. It is usually no more than a gesture. A calm, reassuring response will probably get the upset older person out of the disturbing situation. It often helps to say something like "I'm really sorry that you're so upset, I'm going to do everything I can to help you feel better." Again, the next step is treatment for the relief of these symptoms.

Sexual Delusions

Some delusions are sexual in nature. For example, a man thinks that his wife has become a prostitute and is soliciting all the men in the neighborhood. This is obviously a very difficult problem for the accused spouse to deal with. Since it is usually impossible to dislodge the idea with reasoning (that the wife has always been a faithful partner, the mother of his children, and now a venerable grandmother), the best response is to ignore the accusations and change the subject. As in the other examples of handling disordered thinking, medical supervision is essential, for with the correct medication the mentally impaired older person can be made more comfortable.

Although sexual delusions are not as common as disordered responses to forgotten or misplaced belongings or to paranoid interpretations of things misheard and misperceived, families should be aware of them as a possibility in the process of mental deterioration. The ideas that can be expressed are sometimes bizarre, but you must understand that they simply constitute another symptom of mental impairment.

A dignified, never-married, very elderly woman lawyer complained to her devoted niece that the widower who lived next door had set up some sort of periscope so that he could see her when she undressed and when she used the bathroom. She kept the heavy drapes drawn, but still she knew that the periscope was designed to get around the drapes and into the bathroom. She was so upset by this that she wouldn't take a bath, and she was afraid to change her clothes. Although she had previously been meticulous and proper in her appearance, she now looked and smelled like a derelict. The niece, who had a shared checking account for emergencies, hired a homemaker to care for her aunt, but the aunt sent her away, explaining that she had to protect the housekeeper from the neighbor's periscope. When she complained to the police, they told her to see a doctor. She became agitated, exclaiming that they thought she was crazy but she wasn't. As the aunt became more frail, the niece was able to have her hospitalized for malnutrition and dehydration. After a period of treatment and medication for her delusion, she was able to be discharged home with the supervision of a visiting nurse and home health aide. She never mentioned the neighbor or the periscope again.

Sometimes impaired old people complain that someone is causing strange sensations in their private parts. This person could be someone from the neighborhood—a delivery boy, the letter carrier, the librarian, the landlord; or it could be a celebrity—the mayor, the cardinal, a movie star, even God. The sensations can be sent through wires, antennas, sprays, etc. The possibilities are endless, although there are patterns recognizable to physicians and other health professionals.

We have no idea how such delusions are formed. It is almost incomprehensible that people who have been normal, productive citizens with no history of sexual problems could in old age be troubled by such aberrant experiences. We have to simply accept the fact that it can appear as a symptom when the brain miscarries its signals, and if possible laugh at the incongruity of some of the delusions. One memorable lady in my experience delighted everyone with the wonderful humor with which she excused herself constantly for her missing memory. "Call me Mollie," she'd tell everyone, "I forgot my other name." Mollie was so ugly and shriveled that she was almost a caricature. She was the pet of all the nurses and aides on her floor in the nursing home, and they would take special pains to dress her prettily, always tying her sparse hair with a bright-colored ribbon. One day, out of the blue, Mollie reported to the nurse on her floor that a sheik had come to see her during the night with a bunch of wives, and he wanted her to be part of his harem! "Go away," she screamed, "I'll call the doctor." This went on night after night, and Mollie pleaded with the nurse to do something about it. "When I was young and beautiful," she said, "I was happy when my husband left me alone. What does this sheik want from me now that I'm old and ugly?"

Mollie was reassured of the protection of the nursing staff, and after a while, with the help of some medication, the delusion passed. But everyone on staff who knew Mollie, to whom she repeated her problem, marveled at the activity of the impaired brain and the unlimited range of experience in the secret, personal spaces we all possess.

Is there a lesson here? Not really, because it's all part of a realm of the as yet unknown. We do not know the cause of the particular behavior. We know of no definite relationship to anything in the background of the older person who suffers such indignities. All we can do is understand that it can happen and accept these delusions as we would accept a limp and a cane in someone with a broken hip. Family members must struggle with their embarrassment. Don't be afraid to talk to others about your feelings in this area. You will feel much easier if you can share your sense of shock with others, perhaps even laugh about it, and you may come to see it's not usually a very serious problem.

The Art of Reassurance

Usually the paranoid older person is harmless and does not panic if he is given the opportunity to talk about what's bothering him—without being contradicted. It takes practice, however, to develop the art of responding to a mentally disturbed person. The most important skill is to let him know that you are sorry that something is upsetting him and that you would like to help. You might put your arm around your relative and say, "I can see how upset you are by this, and I wish I could stop what's bothering you, but I don't know what I can do." Or you might say, "I'll see what can be done." Often an expression of concern is enough, because the disturbed older person is usually partially aware that you can't stop the super from sending electrical impulses through the radiators or that others are not able to hear his voices.

Medical Supervision

An important step in caring for a paranoid relative is getting him to see a doctor who might prescribe some medication to control the agitation associated with the disordered thinking. This requires skilled handling, since a suspicious, frightened older person can easily misinterpret your motives in suggesting medical care and include you in his paranoid system. Say that you're concerned that your relative doesn't seem well and you'd like him to see a doctor. It may work if you say that he looks tired or nervous, or perhaps that he is losing weight. Many complaints can be found that can be a legitimate reason for getting him to a doctor.

Ironically, if medication is prescribed for a paranoid patient, it might not be taken if the patient suspects that the doctor is giving him something for a mental condition. But if the doctor says it's something for his nerves, or blood pressure, or appetite, the patient is more likely to take the medication. Sometimes a concerned relative and the doctor can plan a strategy on the best method to get the patient's cooperation. I remember one case in which the relative told the doctor that the impaired old person would take vitamins but not medicine. The doctor told the patient that he was prescribing a special new potent vitamin. The patient was given a tranquilizer and her behavior improved so that she was able to remain at home with the help of her relative.

It may seem unfair and even unethical to lie to someone who is suffering from a mental illness. This dilemma falls into the realm of what professionals call "informed consent." There is increasing concern about ethical issues in medical treatment, with an emphasis on a patient's right to make choices based on full knowledge of his diagnosis and potential results of treatment. Informed consent, however, requires that the patient be *capable of understanding the diagnosis, the treatment, and the consequences of his choices*. Clearly, the mentally impaired older person cannot use the information provided, therefore this right passes to his responsible relative. If you find that you have to invent a fiction in order to provide treatment for a disturbed older person, is it bad? Isn't the old notion of a "white lie" helpful in these circumstances?

To summarize this section, I would like to stress that a paranoid reaction can be viewed as a defense mechanism used by a vulnerable, frightened older person who cannot accept the changes that may be taking place, both within him and in his perception of his environment. The reactions are usually harmless, but at times the older person may panic from his fears and lash out aggressively.

The older person suffering from paranoid ideas is often relieved of the anxieties that produce these beliefs by talking about them, complaining about the problem to whoever is nearby and is viewed as being able to help. But those to whom the complaints are directed are often upset by the obviously irrational ideas and unable to give the sought-for reassurance. Even those who recognize this need, and offer some kind of reassurance at first, become worn out by the ongoing demand for a sympathetic ear or for the sense of help from someone viewed as powerful. The mentally impaired older person with paranoid symptoms should be guided into medical treatment as soon as possible, before everyone who can help becomes alienated or worn out.

8

Other Upsetting Problems

This chapter will discuss some common problems that cause embarrassment and confusion for the relatives of the victims of severe mental deterioration.

INCONTINENCE

One of the most painful changes that can occur in the mentally impaired aged is the loss of their ability to use the toilet by themselves. This does not become a problem for all old people who suffer mental impairment, for the pattern and course of brain failure and its effects on mental and bodily functioning varies from person to person. But for those whose learned behavior of when and where to use the toilet becomes unlearned due to brain damage in the area that controls bladder and bowel function, the emotional impact can be devastating, both to themselves and to those who love and care for them.

There is no condition that is more demoralizing than incontinence. It engenders feelings of shame, helplessness, hopelessness, and even self-hate. Even the most tactful, sensitive handling may not be enough to overcome the depth of despair felt by the older person who has this problem and is at least partially aware of it. And the relative of someone who becomes incontinent has the problem of recognizing his own upset feelings as well as his impaired kin's.

Before accepting urinary and fecal incontinence as one more symptom with which to cope, however, it is important to know that there are many possible causes. For example, if an impaired older person wets himself on the way to the bathroom, it may be that the urge to urinate comes on so quickly and with so much stress that there isn't enough time to get to the bathroom. Incontinence with urgency and frequency may be caused by a urinary tract infection, prostate problems, or other physical difficulties that might be corrected. In view of our discomfort in discussing these bodily functions, it is understandable that when the mentally impaired older person shows the first signs of incontinence, we may react too quickly, failing to make an honest effort to determine whether it is treatable or at least manageable. Far too often this symptom becomes the reason for institutionalizing someone who, if the incontinence could be diagnosed and managed, would be happier and better adjusted outside of an institution.

The first step, then, is to overcome the sense of shame and learn to talk to your relative about the incontinence in a way that will help you gather the facts you'll need if you are to help a physician make as accurate a diagnosis as possible. Find words that will be comfortable for you and your impaired relative, that will avoid expressing disapproval. The word "elimination" is often used for bowel movement and is understood by professionals and lay people. The word "voiding" is sometimes more comfortable to use than "urinating." The important thing is to be understood without getting judgmental or emotional.

Never treat your relative as a bad child. He is not bad, and he is not a child. If you say, "Don't feel upset that you soiled yourself," and "Let's see if we can find out what's wrong," you will probably be clear in conveying your concern. If you are upset by the incident and say something like "How did you manage to soil yourself like that!" you will convey revulsion, obviously the opposite of what is needed.

If your relative's mental functioning is very deteriorated, you will not be able to get much information from him as to why he wasn't able to get to the toilet on time. You will have to look for indirect clues by observing him or having someone else observe him over a period of several days. Sometimes the incontinence is a result of disorientation, when the older person no longer remembers where he is or where the bathroom is. While trying to remember where to go, he may relieve himself wherever he is. Or he may use a closet or a wastebasket because of an urgency to relieve himself. Careful observation of his behavior can help you to anticipate his needs and guide him to the bathroom in time, or train someone else to give this type of care.

If the diagnosis determines that your relative will have

a chronic problem with incontinence, you must be prepared for drastic changes. If the incontinent person is your spouse and you are used to a double bed, you may find it more practical to switch to twin beds or separate rooms. It is not easy to manage incontinence at home, but it can be done with the assumption of new roles and new skills.

Medical supply stores can advise you about bed pads to protect the mattress, commodes to use next to a bed, and adult-size diapers and waterproof pants. But they cannot prepare you for the actual problem of changing soiled and wet pants and cleaning the private areas of your dear one.

Nurses and aides who are responsible for the personal care and hygiene of older persons require special training. Some are better suited to this than others by virtue of their personalities and temperaments. The same holds true for relatives who perform this very personal service. All can use some special training (perhaps from a visiting nurse) in the skills required to toilet and clean an incontinent, mentally impaired older person. But all will not be successful, either because of temperament or because of an inability to act like a nurse or aide instead of a daughter, son, wife, or husband.

Most of our behavior is learned through roles in life. We learn how to juggle the rules and obligations that come with our many roles so that they fit together as comfortably as possible. If someone tries to meet the responsibilities of too many roles at the same time, he will find himself under too much stress. The sociologists call this *role strain*. In order to manage these many roles with the least strain, it is necessary to come up with a realistic agenda of what you can do. Therefore, if you are thinking of taking on the role of care-giver to an elderly relative who has become incontinent, you must learn some of the skills of a nurse or aide and try to anticipate whether these new tasks fit into the set of all your other roles. This new role would include training yourself to attend to the new needs of your impaired kin, such as when and how to take him to the toilet, how to put on and take off protective garments if they're needed (such as pads and waterproof underpants), and how to protect the bed and other furniture.

If you feel you have the patience and temperament to fit this into your normal schedule, there is still a very big hurdle to consider. When you assume a new role, your relative must also be able to *accept* your new role and change his behavior accordingly. Many mentally impaired older persons are not able to understand the need for changing their behavior. With incontinence you will be dealing with such massive embarrassment and even denial of the problem, that it may be very difficult for you to assume your new role, no matter how sensitively you handle it.

If you can overcome these obstacles and provide this care for your relative without excessive strain, you can experience great satisfaction. But if you can't manage it after all, don't feel guilty for seeking the help of a nursing home. The nursing home may be much better equipped and staffed to provide this level of care, and your embarrassed relative may find it more acceptable to receive care from a detached professional than from someone who is emotionally close.

HYGIENE

One of the saddest signs of mental impairment in a previously normal old person is a lack of attention to personal hygiene. When the impaired old person denies the need for personal care and refuses help, it often causes a feeling of panic on the part of the caring relatives. There is a sense of shame, both for the older person who is no longer clean and neat looking, and for the responsible relatives, fearing that people will think they're not taking proper care of their kin.

If your relative denies that he needs care, try to figure out why bathing, grooming, and dressing appropriately have become so difficult. To do this you must first overcome your own embarrassment and recognize whether you are feeling angry with your relative or yourself. A failure to acknowledge your feelings about this will interfere with your ability to analyze why this has become a problem.

Remember that when memory loss is very advanced and messages for old automatic skills are no longer available from the brain, the routine acts of bathing, dressing, and grooming become very complex operations. Even deciding what to wear can become an overwhelming challenge. The purpose of bathing may be forgotten, or the mechanics of taking a bath may be too difficult. Assess just what is making it difficult for your relative to dress and bathe appropriately, and develop your own techniques for helping your kin in this sensitive area.

If your kin is very stubborn and uncooperative despite your efforts, perhaps it will help to ask yourself whether your standards are too high. Remember how fashions and fads change—the proper length and style of hair, the length of skirts, slacks for women, blue jeans for businessmen and professionals. I remember how stubborn my father became when we tried to persuade him to shave every day. When we gave up and his beard grew in, we found that Dad looked rather distinguished.

Even standards of cleanliness vary, although there is a generally held norm that makes most people comfortable in terms of health, sanitation, and inoffensiveness to others. If your relative is absolutely refusing a bath or sponge bath, and if his lack of hygiene is intolerable, his doctor might prescribe some medication to ease the anxiety that is probably contributing to his behavior. If the doctor feels that a tranquilizer is necessary to help with this problem, there will need to be extra vigilance to prevent an accident that might result from the unaccustomed relaxation. The principle to follow in supervising the personal hygiene of your mentally impaired kin is to develop greater tolerance but be as protective as necessary. Search for the balance that will satisfy your needs as well as your relative's and the community's, with the least damage to all.

INAPPROPRIATE SEXUAL BEHAVIOR

When damage occurs in the center of the brain that controls sexual impulses, the impaired older person might display sexual behavior that can be extremely upsetting to others. (The idea of *any* sexual activity in older people can be upsetting to some relatives. Consider the following observation by comedian Sam Levenson: When he first learned about sex, he said he could believe it about his father, maybe, but his mother? *Never!*) Because old people are seen as parent figures, their children may have difficulty thinking of them as having sexual needs.

It is not surprising, therefore, that when a mentally impaired older person displays uninhibited sexuality, it can cause distress to those around him.

Sometimes the sexual behavior is the innocent consequence of the older person's impaired memory, confusion, or disorientation, as illustrated in the following example.

Mrs. Mahler was divorced and living with her two small children when her mother died. Her father, who had had a stroke, had been very dependent upon her mother and was unable to live alone. Mrs. Mahler moved him into her apartment and set up a place for him to sleep in the living room. Weeks passed, and the family tried to adjust to the new arrangements. One night Mrs. Mahler awoke to find that her father had crept into her bed and was fondling her sexually. She panicked and became hysterical, unable to recognize that her father had forgotten where he was and that his wife had died, and that he thought he was getting into bed with his wife. Her father also became very upset, although he was confused about the incident. Mrs. Mahler was so disturbed by the episode that she was no longer able to care for him or even to relate to him as she had previously. She arranged for a nursing home admission as quickly as she could. Although she could understand intellectually that her father's sexual behavior was harmless and not intentionally directed at her, she was emotionally unable to overcome her feelings of disgust.

This case points up the depth of our feelings when sexual taboos are violated. It takes a great deal of understanding and discussion to get over our upset feelings when the mentally impaired old man or woman we are concerned about is no longer able to conform to normal sexual mores. As in other problem behaviors, it must be seen as a symptom of mental impairment. But when the most fundamental taboos are forgotten, it is more difficult to accept the offending behavior as symptomatic.

Fortunately, inappropriate sexual behavior is not a problem in most mentally impaired aged, but when it does occur, it is often experienced as degenerate and degrading. Frequently the behavior takes the form of masturbation in public or handling of genitalia without awareness of the presence of others. If those who witness this behavior can understand that although there are deeply ingrained negative feelings about masturbation, it is not considered an abnormal or immoral act by most mental health professionals, they might be less inclined to overreact. It should be viewed as resulting from a loss in inhibition about the requirement of privacy. The appropriate response would be to distract the older person from what he is doing and get him to a private area.

Sometimes an increase in sexual activity is a reaction to anxiety or even to depression. This should be discussed with the older person's physician, for if emotional symptoms are indeed the cause of the inappropriate sexual expressions, then they can be treated with medication, leading to a reduction of the sexual behavior.

Sometimes the uninhibited older person may make upsetting sexual remarks or advances. Although it can be shocking to hear vulgar and suggestive language from a previously polite, discreet person, it is best to handle this lightly, with humor, or even by ignoring the behavior.

We do not know why this particular behavior occurs in some and not in others. There is no known relation to a person's past sexual experiences. It should be viewed simply as one more change that can occur with advancing mental impairment.

When the older person still has the privacy of his own home or the home of a relative, the inappropriate sexual behavior need be understood only by the few persons who are responsible for his care. However, if he goes for walks unsupervised in the neighborhood, his sexual behavior can cause serious disturbances. Care must be taken to protect the older person whose judgment is failing from wandering without supervision outside his home, both for his own safety and dignity and for the comfort and protection of others. If sexual behavior occurs outside the home, the person who is supervising should remove the impaired older person from the embarrassing situation and, if there is time, explain that the behavior is caused by mental impairment.

Occasionally, mentally impaired older persons who are in the protective setting of a nursing home also display overt sexual behavior. How this is handled depends very much on the skills of the nursing home staff and the level of training they have had in understanding this behavior.

In some ways it can be more difficult to manage the inappropriate behavior in an institution because of the lack of privacy. Often the staffs in nursing homes, despite their training, display a leering attitude and make fun of the older person displaying such behavior. Institutional staffs must be exposed to in-service training about sexuality in old age, understanding it as a normal drive and understanding as well the special problems posed when mental impairment leads to loss of judgment and inhibitions. Nursing home employees are sometimes subject to sexual advances and they must learn to recognize these as a sign of the patient's inability to control impulsive behavior and to judge what is inappropriate. They must also learn, just as family members must learn, to understand their own strong feelings about sexuality and the aged, and they must learn the techniques of distracting the impaired older person from the sexual behavior and getting him to a more private area.

The staff must also exercise vigilance to protect against the exercise of socially inappropriate behavior, as when an impaired older person gets into bed with another confused patient. Although the experience may in fact be pleasant for both parties, the important issue is that the patients would not indulge in this public behavior if they were mentally intact. This calls for a protective attitude on the part of the staff to prevent upsetting both the patients and their families.

There has been much public discussion in recent years about the sexual needs and rights of institutional residents. This has centered on the needs of mentally normal persons who can handle their sexuality privately if they have the opportunity to do so. This is not applicable to the needs of the mentally impaired aged, who may no longer be able to distinguish between private and public areas and whose loss of inhibition may lead to indiscreet behavior. The mentally impaired patients first need protection, then privacy.

This chapter has dealt with some of the most disturbing problems that may confront you as the relative of an impaired older person. By recognizing your emotions in dealing with them, and by talking about your feelings with anyone who can share them, you will find it easier to cope. If you remember that these behaviors are symptoms of mental impairment and that your relative cannot change his behavior through understanding and reason, you will be able to develop your own skills in handling the problems. Don't give up on searching for solutions. Your relative's condition will not remain constant—the circumstances will change, and you must be prepared to change with them.

9

The Paradox
of Medications

M any people have strong
feelings about drugs or
medications. Some avoid taking any, even when they're
medically necessary. Some demand them even when the
doctor doesn't recommend any. These contrasting attitudes are found not only among the general population
but among professionals in the health field as well. There
are some doctors who will prescribe drugs freely for every
complaint, such as nervousness, sleeplessness, or tired-
ness. There are some, however, who prescribe very few
drugs.

Why should there be such differences in attitudes and

practice? And how do these different beliefs affect the mentally impaired aged patient?

This chapter will examine the issues concerning the medicating of the mentally impaired aged. The discussion will be concerned largely with the drugs prescribed for mental and behavioral problems for those older persons whose mental impairment has been diagnosed as chronic, although, since the elderly are frequently medicated for other conditions, some attention will be paid to these medications as well.

The majority of drugs now used for mental conditions have been available only since the mid-1950s, and the most effective medications are for *depression, anxiety, agitation*, and *thought disorders*. However, all of these medications require careful monitoring since they all have some potential side effects that may be uncomfortable or even dangerous. The challenge to the physician and the responsible family is to find the medication that presents the least risk and still can effectively ease the upsetting mental symptoms.

DEPRESSION

The most common mental disorder in old age is depression, which has been described also in chapter 3. It is no surprise that depression affects an older person who becomes aware of his deteriorating mental abilities. This is called a *reactive depression*, since it is in reaction to a problem beyond the control of the older person. A very normal reaction to a very serious problem, this depression can be treated even when the other mental losses may be irreversible.

There are, though, several obstacles that may keep an older person from being medicated appropriately for depression. First, the doctor may assume that the symptoms are part of the total symptoms of chronic organic brain syndrome, and therefore not treatable. Next, if the doctor does decide to try an antidepressant, he must choose among several types and many brands, such as Tofranil, Pertofrane, Elavil, Nardil, Marplan, and Parnak. There then has to be careful monitoring, with feedback to the doctor on the reaction of the older person so that the dosage can be modified, if necessary, or the medication changed altogether. This requires both a genuine interest on the part of the doctor and a generosity about the time needed for discussing the effects of the drug.

A common error in prescribing for the older person involves the dosage selected for a particular drug. Most recommended dosages are geared to an "average person" who is usually of average weight and young to middle-aged. The depressed older person may be underweight, since lack of appetite can accompany depression, or overweight, since inactivity is also common. These factors would sharply influence the size of the dosage of effective medication. Furthermore, the older person's changing physiology causes drugs to be absorbed and utilized differently from the way they might be in a younger person. As noted, this is due to slower liver and kidney function as well as to changes in the heart, lungs, and circulatory system. In addition, in the older person there may be a higher proportion of body fat where drugs might be stored when not excreted normally. It is obvious why many errors might occur in prescribing for an older person even when he appears to be functioning normally.

Even if the medication is prescribed and is being taken in the correct dosage, there can still be detours on the road to effective treatment. Many antidepressants take up to three or four weeks to be effective. The older person who continues to feel depressed for weeks may become discouraged and refuse to continue with the medication. Or the family supervising the medication regimen may discontinue it after a few weeks if it is unaware of the period of time required for the effects to be seen.

There are also side effects to be considered. Some old people may develop dry mouth, nasal congestion, constipation, urinary retention, and sexual impotence in response to an antidepressant. Many antidepressants cause drowsiness or dizziness because of a drop in blood pressure, and this can lead to falls. Some can cause irregular heartbeat, blurred vision, and eye pain. In some old persons there can be a toxic effect that causes hallucinations. I remember two different residents of a nursing home who saw cats when they took Tofranil! The cats disappeared when the drug was discontinued.

Sometimes the antidepressant medication has an opposite effect to that which is intended (called a paradoxical reaction), and increases the depression instead of lessening it. Other times it can worsen the symptoms of mental confusion and disorientation.

With all of these potential adverse effects, you can understand why some doctors hesitate even to start a patient on such a medication regimen, or why they may discontinue it at the very first report of an unpleasant side effect. The knowledgeable family should report any of these complaints and should not be shy about asking the doctor to try another medication if he does not suggest it himself. Sometimes three or four different medications of varying strengths must be tried before one is found that will help.

Of course, treating depression with medication is no

substitute for contact with concerned people, but the relief produced by the medications can make it easier for the older person to respond to the concerned people around him (if his degree of brain failure permits). In this respect, the purpose of drugs is to minimize the degree of infirmity that is affecting the mentally impaired older person.

A very important area for family vigilance is awareness of any alcohol that the older person might be consuming. While moderate use of alcohol is considered helpful in maintaining good health in a relatively alert older person, it can be very harmful to someone who is mentally impaired. Wine, beer, or hard liquor can have very serious interactions with medications, especially antidepressants and sedatives. Check with the pharmacist or physician for advice about mixing medications and alcohol.

Despite the obstacles to effective treatment—the resistance of the older person, the pessimism of the doctor, the discomfort of potential side effects, and even the danger involved—with close supervision and correct dosages, very marked improvement in mood can be achieved through medication. Do not give up too soon. With enough experimentation and careful management, depression can be relieved.

ANXIETY REACTIONS

It is quite normal for people to feel anxious or fearful about many of life's events. Some deal with their anxieties more easily than others. As people age, they become more vulnerable to the threatening events of life, and at the same time their abilities to cope with these events may become less effective. Handling emotions calls for a healthy physiology and a responsive central nervous system.

When an older person who is also mentally impaired becomes anxious or frightened about events that he may or may not perceive accurately, his reaction can be extreme. The anxiety reaction of a mentally impaired older person might be expressed in agitated behavior. He might pace the floor, unable to sit quietly. He might fidget nervously, restlessly. He might constantly rummage through the house or his room or his bureau drawers, needing to be busy, using up the nervous energy created by the state of anxiety. He might wander through the house, or outside the house, getting lost. He might respond irritably to whoever is near. He might shout, scream, push, spit, curse, kick, or hit with objects (such as canes), all in response to what appears to be threatening.

All of these behaviors can be helped by the correct dosage of the appropriate medication, usually some form of tranquilizer. But often, as soon as the word "tranquilizer" comes up, there is a negative reaction—another anxiety reaction, this one holding that tranquilizers turn you into a mindless zombie. As a result, many behaviors that reflect the extreme mental discomfort of the older person are tolerated without attempts to modify or treat the behavior. This failure to medicate is just as harmful as overmedicating.

When the anxiety reaction is caused by a temporary situation, such as moving to a new environment, which should clear up as an adjustment is made, minor tranquilizers are sometimes given, usually Librium or Valium. These should be prescribed for a limited period and in the lowest effective dosage, since they are potentially dangerous for older people (they can accumulate in the system and cause a dependency on the drug). Additionally, when the older person is mentally frail, these drugs can cause further mental impairment.

When a mentally impaired old person exhibits acutely anxious behavior, the drugs of choice are usually the so-called major tranquilizers, such as Thorazine, Mellaril, Haldol, and Stelazine. If the patient is both depressed and agitated due to anxiety, Sinequan or Elavil might be prescribed.

Although all of these drugs can relieve symptoms of anxiety, they all have side effects that can cause other symptoms. And some of the symptoms may seem worse than the one that is being treated.

The most common of the side effects caused by the major tranquilizers are symptoms that are similar to those of Parkinson's disease: rigidity of the muscles, muscle weakness, and tremors that look like palsy. The older person may become uncontrollably restless. His muscles may become uncoordinated, causing facial tics and grimaces. The muscles that control the tongue and other organs of speech may be impaired and he may have difficulty speaking and swallowing. Less common but perhaps even more upsetting, he may develop spasms that stiffen his body into an arch, with only his head and feet touching the bed, or spasms that contract the neck muscles so that his head twists to one side.

In addition, he may be troubled by some of the same side effects as those triggered by antidepressant medications: dry mouth, constipation, urinary retention, nasal congestion, sleepiness, and listlessness.

All of these symptoms will stop if the medication that triggered them is discontinued. Since there is no way at present of predicting how any medication will affect a particular person, finding a helpful drug regimen is more of an art than a science—a matter of trial and error. The motto should be "Do it until you get it right." It may be very frightening to see someone you love stiffen up and start to shake with tremors, or speak as though he's drunk, but these are only temporary reactions. Call the doctor for a change in medication.

Occasionally a patient who has been taking a major tranquilizer for some time develops a condition of involuntary and bizarre movements of his lips, tongue, and jaw (tardive dyskinesia), which does not always clear up when the medication is discontinued. It was found recently, however, that lecithin (a food substance sold in health-food stores) seems to be effective in treating these upsetting movements.

Unfortunately, sometimes the original symptoms get worse with the medication and the doctors increase the dosage instead of changing the medication. You have to monitor the effects of the dosages closely and report back quickly. Remember, there are relatively few doctors who are specialized in geriatrics or the medical care of the aged, and few are interested enough in the aged to have developed the skills of psychopharmacology (the science of drug treatment of mental disorders) as these relate to the elderly. Therefore, if you become aware of some of the benefits as well as the side effects of medication and raise questions with the doctor about treating your kin's disturbed behavior with drugs, you should be able to judge whether he is interested enough to use the trial-and-error method effectively.

Sometimes, when a patient develops Parkinsonian symptoms, as described earlier, the doctor will add anti-Parkinson's drugs to the regimen rather than change the dosage or the medication. This practice should be questioned. In fact you, the responsible relative, have a right and a duty to question, to request medication, and to refuse medication on behalf of your impaired kin. If the doctor is too authoritarian to accept your questions, you may want to search for another doctor who is more understanding.

In medicating for anxiety, another area of concern is the use of sedatives for people who cannot sleep at night. Expert opinion holds that sleeping medication, such as sedatives or hypnotics, can be very harmful for all elderly people and particularly so for the mentally impaired person whose brain function may be very marginal. The effects of a nighttime sedative usually carry over into the daytime, because the drug is not excreted sufficiently in an old person. This causes an even greater level of impairment. It is considered better geriatric practice to prescribe a larger dose of an anti-anxiety medication or a major tranquilizer to be given at night to help the older person sleep without risking the sedative effects during the day.

Still another possibility to be alert to is that Thorazine-type medications can worsen existing depression. If you notice that your anxious relative appears more depressed after starting on Thorazine, be sure to mention it to the doctor and ask if it is a side effect that should be treated.

PHYSICIANS' ATTITUDES

It is a very difficult task to become a partner, even a junior partner, in the medical treatment of your kin. Most physicians are trained to take full responsibility for their patients' treatment. They take full credit for cures and full responsibility for failure. Perhaps this is why many doctors act as if they believe that patients (and their representatives) should trust the doctor's judgment completely and follow his orders unquestioningly. Perhaps they are more afraid of the failures than they care to admit, and they cover up this fear with a mystique about their procedures and a reluctance to share information.

"What's my blood pressure, Doctor?" "Don't worry about it. If there was anything wrong, I would tell you." This exchange probably sounds familiar to many readers. It typifies the attitude that you should just relax and put yourself in the doctor's care.

Well, that often works. But when it comes to the intricacies of diagnosing and treating the aged, and particularly the mentally impaired aged, the doctor *must* enlist the cooperation of the family. And if he is not aware of his need for family cooperation in effective treatment, you must try to clarify your role to him, tactfully but assertively.

Doctors are highly trained and extremely skilled, but they are also human beings, with their own anxieties and defenses. They are also creatures of habit, preferring to follow patterns of treatment that are familiar to them rather than experimenting. For example, a doctor may prescribe Thorazine routinely for a full range of agitated behaviors. If after a period of time the behavior is still upsetting, and a relative asks if Haldol or Stelazine might help, the doctor may feel defensive and resist changing medications. The question is, how long should a trial of medication continue before something else is tried? The family has the right to ask questions and to expect a willingness on the part of the doctor to keep trying until the right dosage of the right medication is found.

I remember an incident with an elderly couple who lived in a retirement community where medical care was available as part of the services. The husband became very agitated as part of a deteriorating mental condition and would disturb other residents in the communal dining room. The doctor prescribed some medication, but it didn't help. He increased the dosage, but the symptoms worsened. The wife, also elderly, was unable to handle his behavior, and two daughters who lived nearby came daily to help. But the behavior continued to be upsetting—he was shouting, pushing people, even throwing dishes. Eventually the management of the retirement community told the family that there was nothing that could help him, and they were given notice that they had to move him to a nursing home. The medical staff took the position that his condition had become unmanageable, and that medication could not control it. Finally the daughters arranged to have their father hospitalized.

After several weeks the daughters reported that the hospital had tried several medications and finally found one that was effective, but the medical staff of the retirement community could not believe that the hospital had succeeded where they had failed. They took a firm stand with the administrator that the resident should not be allowed to return to his apartment. The daughters smuggled him in somehow, and to the embarrassment of the medical staff, the resident was indeed calm and happy to be back with his wife. On the correct maintenance dosage of the right medication, he managed to be a model resident for many years.

This example shows how even experienced professionals are subject to biases about treatment and can make mistakes. What can you do when confronted by a stalemate with medical opinion? If you are not satisfied that everything which might help has been tried, get another opinion. But remember to be realistic in your expectations.

These medications can ease agitation, with its restless or otherwise upsetting behaviors, but they cannot reverse the brain failure that your relative is experiencing.

OBSTACLES TO GIVING MEDICATIONS

Some old people are not used to taking medications. They may not even be able to swallow an aspirin or they may no longer be able to swallow pills. If they are confused, they may not understand why they should take the pills. If they are suspicious, they may be afraid to take the pills.

The family must try to anticipate its relative's attitude toward taking medications. You may have to ask the doctor to prescribe something in liquid form, preferably tasteless, that can be put into another beverage, or something that can be crushed and mixed with applesauce or mashed banana. Use your ingenuity and knowledge of your relative's likes and dislikes to figure out how to get him to take the medication.

Finally, remember that your relative may be very sensitive about the reasons he is taking medication. If you can find a plausible explanation—"for your blood pressure" or "to help you feel less nervous" or "to build up your strength"—it will make things easier all around. Whatever reason works for your relative is the one to try. If you feel guilty about lying to your relative, he may sense your discomfort and refuse the medication. Train yourself to focus on the necessity for the medication, which is to achieve a more comfortable state for your relative; this should alleviate your guilt and help you accomplish your task.

ETHICAL DILEMMAS

As we have discussed in the earlier chapter on paranoid behavior, underlying your uncomfortable feelings in handling the medication needs of your anxious, agitated relative with less than absolute honesty is the conflict with basic social values that teach us to be truthful and forthright in all relationships. Democratic values emphasize the rights of the individual, and one of those rights is the right to be informed about medical treatment.

But rights carry certain responsibilities. The mentally impaired older person usually has lost the capacity to understand his behavior, and consequently the need to modify it. Of what value is it to insist that your mentally impaired relative be informed as to what medication is being given and what its purpose is, if, as a result, he refuses the medication?

Those who object to the ethics of medicating people without their full knowledge and consent usually see it as a form of social control imposed on an unwilling recipient—a kind of totalitarianism. (The term "chemical straitjacket" came about to describe a condition of medication control that restricts someone's freedom.) These objections are valid if medications are used improperly, without attempting to find the right drug or the correct dosage. (The classic objections refer to those nursing-home patients who sit "doped up" all day long in front of a TV, or in depressing surroundings with no activities. This does not usually occur in well-run nursing homes, and there is no reason to tolerate it in any home. This will be discussed in detail in chapter 11, which deals with nursing homes.)

It is important to recognize that some professionals go to extremes in their concern to avoid "chemical straitjackets." Because of their strong convictions that it is unethical to modify someone's behavior by medication without their informed consent, they will tolerate behavior that reflects extreme stress both for the patient and for those who are caring for him. Perhaps this is a result of viewing an ethical principle in the abstract rather than taking a philosophical approach that emphasizes the humane needs of the impaired individual and those close to him.

But many others avoid medication because of a realistic concern for adverse side effects. As a result, you may find patients in nursing homes who scream constantly for no apparent physical reason, or who roam incessantly, making life intolerable for roommates and visitors. The staff seems to be able to "tune out" and not pay attention to these cries for help. It is astonishing that professionals who would routinely order medications to relieve *physical* pain sometimes are inattentive to *psychic* pain.

One can legitimately question whether the reason for not calming these agitated patients with drugs is related to ethical principles, to a concern about side effects, or to unwillingness to give the time necessary to try out medications until the right one is found. My personal experience leads me to believe that too often both overmedicating and undermedicating reflect the unwillingness of the health team to give the time needed to individualize the treatment. The knowledgeable family can change this pattern.

If your relative is disturbed and still living in the community, you yourself may hold out against medicating him out of a sense of guilt that one reason for tranquilizing him is to keep him from driving everyone else crazy. You may feel still more guilty if, as a result of the medication, your relative gets dizzy and falls or develops other side effects. But you should be able to overcome your feelings of guilt if you recognize that the purpose of the medication is, first and foremost, to relieve the anxieties or disordered thoughts that make your relative so agitated. It is a humane goal to try to make a disturbed older person more comfortable.

EXPERIMENTAL DRUGS

New knowledge about the nature of mental impairment has led to experiments with a large number of substances to try to improve brain function, particularly memory. The use of vasodilators (such as Hydergine), which should increase the amount of oxygen to the brain by dilating the blood vessels, has been studied for some years. The results have been inconclusive to date. It is felt that Hydergine may help to improve the metabolism of brain cells and thereby increase the amount of oxygen for patients with mental impairment of the Alzheimer's type, but it does not appear to help the mentally impaired with multi-infarct dementia, whose blood vessels may lack elasticity.

Lecithin (which contains the B-complex vitamin choline) may increase the amount of acetylcholine in the brain, a neurotransmitter involved in memory. Most of the studies done with very impaired persons indicate no improvement, but there may be improvement in people in the early stages of memory loss.

There are many promising new drugs that effect the metabolism of the brain or improve neurotransmitter activity, but thus far the studies have not included sufficient samples of people in varying stages of mental impairment. Therefore, at present, the families of the mentally impaired aged cannot look to drugs for hope in symptom improvement, but only for symptom relief.

This chapter has called for a large measure of involvement from the concerned family, perhaps more than can be reasonably expected.

Just remember that no health professional knows your relative as well as you do. The doctor should welcome your observations and questions as a contribution to better care of his patient. Unfortunately, many doctors will not understand your role. If you feel that this is true in your case and that it interferes with good care, you should try to find another doctor. If you don't have the energy to accomplish this, don't let it add to your burden. You can do only as much as possible with a limited amount of time and energy.

Most important—be aware of the attitudes and biases that may be influencing the decision to medicate or not. The principle of minimum intervention is a sound one in good geriatric care, leading to a lessened possibility of harm. But the minimum of treatment should be adequate for the needs of the impaired old person. Be sure that your relative is treated as an individual, and that every attempt is made to relieve the sorrow, bewilderment, rage, or terror of his impaired mental condition.

10

*The Paradox
of Institutional Care*

*A*s mental impairment gets worse, many families find themselves in conflict about whether or not to consider institutional care for their kin, and the need to make a decision about placement sometimes causes panic. Old resentments and rivalries can be rekindled. The decision to institutionalize is experienced psychologically as a final separation. The prospect of separation may start a process of deep sadness and grief, in recognition of a decline that will end only with death. In view of such feelings, and the painful preparation for loss, is institutional care ever preferable to family care?

The significant issue to consider is that of why some families keep their mentally impaired loved ones at home while others place their relatives in nursing homes or similar institutions. Are there factors in the structure of the family that influence these decisions? What role is played by the family's financial circumstances? How is the decision-making process affected by the physical environment or the resources available to help with care? A review of all these elements should provide you with a broader understanding of what we know and what we don't know about family strength when it is challenged by mental impairment in old age.

WHAT IS A FAMILY?

If someone asked you to list the members of your family, whom would you include? Husband, wife, children? Parents? Brothers, sisters? Grandparents, nieces, nephews, aunts, uncles, cousins? Half-brothers and -sisters? Step-brothers and stepsisters? Those who live under one roof? Those on whom you can count in time of trouble? You can see there may be other considerations than mere relationship by blood or marriage.

People of different cultures have different views on who is considered part of their family and who is expected to be available in time of need. But do we really know who shares a particular culture, or do we tend to accept stereotyped notions about groups? Think of a specific ethnic group as an example. Do we know how they feel about family cohesiveness?

First we must identify whether we mean those who are American-born or foreign-born. If foreign-born, are their attitudes conditioned by what part of their country they come from? We must ask if they are religious or not, and, if religious, of which denomination. Each of these attributes can influence the attitudes of the group.

Then we must ask whether we're talking about working class, middle class, professionals, or upper class. Only then can we start to see what the shared attitudes of a specific segment of a particular cultural group might be.

Remember, too, that people of similar cultures may have different views from one generation to the next, as well as from one economic level to another.

Let's test our assumptions with a culture we probably all have some ideas about. What is the position of the aged in the Japanese family? I think that most people would say that the Japanese aged enjoy a favorable status, because of cultural adherence to the ideal of filial piety, or respect for elders.

Sometimes our assumptions seem to be formed like the fable about the blind men and the elephant, in which each man believes the elephant to look like the part he happens to touch, since none of the men can see the whole animal. Some people studying the aged in modern Japan have found that they continue to enjoy the revered status of the past, even though their society is now a highly technological one, with different life-styles for the family. And yet some years ago a Japanese film called *Tokyo Story* was made, which showed the tragedy of an elderly couple that expected to live with their oldest son and his wife. The kinds of apartments available in modern Tokyo made it very inconvenient for the old couple to stay with them, and since both son and daughter-in-law were very busy with their work, they had no time for the parents. Brothers and sisters and in-laws fought with one another as this problem was repeated at the home of each child, leaving the parents mournfully aware of the difference between old cultural ideals and the reality of modern life.

Further support for the discrepancy between family values and family behavior can be inferred from the Japanese nickname for a grandmother, which is *tarai maweshi*. This is taken from the name of a circus act in which a juggler twirls a basket on top of a long pole, passing it while twirling to another pole, where it keeps spinning— the image of the grandmother who is passed from one family member's home to another. It is certainly not an image of filial piety.

So you see, even in the case of a culture about which our assumptions are widely shared, they are not necessarily accurate.

It should be obvious that you can't generalize about which family members can count on one another for different kinds of help, given these possible variations, and yet most of us seem to make certain assumptions about what the family should or should not do for one another. Even the government bases policy decisions on what social services are needed on generalized assumptions of what families should or should not do for one another rather than on what families can or cannot do, or will or will not do.

Attention to how we talk about our families can give us a clue to a source of some of the conflict we experience when an elderly relative needs care. When a middle-aged or older person feels the strain of providing care to an impaired parent, someone might ask, "What about your own family?" By "your own family" is often meant your immediate family—your spouse and children. What does this tell us about the position of the older generations when they become dependent? Is an elderly parent no longer "your own family"? The alert elderly parent may himself say to a concerned adult son or daughter, "Don't worry about me. You have your own family to think about." This is an expression of the cultural assumption that when someone marries, his or her primary responsibilities shift to spouse and children.

Despite the apparent conflicts, most help needed by impaired old people is provided by their families. If they are married, the burden falls primarily on the spouse. If they are widowed, someone in the family usually assumes the responsibility either for direct care or for making sure that care is provided. But given the structure of the modern family and the length of time that the need for care goes on, the kind of help that is provided is not necessarily the best.

Modern times have brought drastic changes in family structure. The most significant ones in terms of the problems with which we are concerned in this book are the unprecedented numbers of people living to very old age, the decrease in family size due to changing birth rates, the revolutionary increase in the number of married women who work outside the home, the increased rate of divorce, and the degree of geographic movement of many members of the family. These changes explain why there are fewer members of a family available to provide care at the time when the older relatives may require it.

And yet, in spite of the availability of fewer potential care-givers, most care that is provided is family care, which is an indication of why there is so much strain and burden experienced by relatives of the mentally impaired aged during these periods of long-term care. Given this phenomenon, it seems unfair that the modern family is criticized for neglecting the aged.

Those who blame the family hold the opinion that its members are alienated from one another, leaving the elderly alone and isolated. Studies of family helping patterns have found that the aged are not isolated, at least not geographically. They usually live near at least one family member with whom regular contact is maintained. This tells us nothing about the *quality* of relationships, however, which may or may not be emotionally satisfying. If family relationships do not provide the warmth and real intimacy that come from shared values and experiences, they cannot be satisfying to all members. But that is not the same as alienation and neglect. (What can be done to enhance the quality of family relationships for those who feel dissatisfied is a serious challenge to our social organization, but it is beyond the scope of this discussion.) The fact remains that in spite of a structure that may make it more difficult for family members to meet one another's expectations of genuine caring, most families continue to behave responsibly toward their elderly. The myth of family neglect serves only to place additional stress on the relatives who assume the burden of care for the impaired aged.

FINANCES

The role of the cost of care and its effect on family finances is sometimes overlooked in understanding why some families place impaired kin in institutions and others do not. This is an extremely complex issue, but it is important to understand the economic factors that can sometimes make the decision for you.

In 1965, Medicare was signed into law as a means of helping older people meet the cost of health care, and

Medicaid became the system for paying for medical care for poor people of all ages. Volumes have been written analyzing the unexpected effect that these two medical payment systems have had on increasing the cost of health care. For our purpose we need only look at a few indicators of the costs to see what impact they may have had on the aged and their families.

From 1965 to about 1975, the monthly cost of nursing-home care in New York City was allowed to rise from approximately $500 to $1,500. It has more than doubled since that time. Since most old people can't afford to pay these rates, and since Medicare does not pay for long-term custodial care, those who need this level of care have to use up almost all of their assets before becoming eligible for Medicaid, which then pays the nursing home its approved rate. Although Medicare was welcomed as a right by older people, regardless of their income level, Medicaid was viewed negatively, like welfare. As a result, many people who might need nursing-home care avoid it because the cost would force them to turn to Medicaid for help.

In the case of the mentally impaired, decisions about money are generally made by their kin. In families with considerable assets, relatives may not want to see their inheritance quickly used up on nursing-home care. On the other hand, a poor working-class family might need every penny of the older person's social security to meet costs of rent and food and might therefore not consider nursing-home placement even if the older person is left alone all day without care or supervision. This type of neglect is more widespread than is generally recognized, and even passes as "family care." One thing that makes me angry is that families are usually praised for maintaining impaired older relatives at home, without any awareness of whether they are providing the kind of care that is needed.

When the mentally impaired older person has a spouse, the cost of care is even more of a factor in determining whether a nursing home is an option. Although Medicaid is a federal program, its regulations vary from state to state, and some states are less liberal than others in providing adequate nursing home care. According to the most recent federal regulations in 1983, when a spouse is institutionalized for more than one month, the income of the spouse in the community is not counted in establishing Medicaid eligibility for nursing home care. However, local Departments of Social Services often ignore these regulations and deny eligibility on the ground of excess resources. Such denials should be appealed by means of requesting a fair hearing. Furthermore, often the spouse in the community depends upon the joint family income to manage, thus most spouses are forced to care for their mentally impaired partners at home, even when it is beyond their physical and emotional capacity.

Economics is certainly not the only factor that makes it difficult to place a spouse in a nursing home, but it can be a crucial one. If this is not recognized, there can be a false idealization of the family that cares for its severely impaired kin at home, adding to the guilt of those who do not.

It is the middle-class family with moderate assets for whom the cost of care is the greatest hardship. Those who have adequate finances obviously can provide themselves with the extra help needed to manage the impaired older person at home, if they can handle it emotionally. And those who are poor enough to be eligible can get some help at home paid for by Medicaid (although usually not as much as is needed), or total help through placement in a nursing home. But those with a moderate income are often hardest hit by these problems, since they are generally afraid to spend as much as is necessary to obtain the amount of care required.

Very often, older people may be eligible for Medicaid and supplementary security income (SSI), which would enable them to obtain care while still in the community, but they don't know how to go about getting it. Information about applications can be obtained from a local Social Security office or through the Department of Health and Human Resources. However, older people may be embarrassed to let others know what a marginal income they have, or they may be unable to follow through on instructions regarding application procedures. They may travel to the Medicaid office and find that they don't have the papers needed to verify their age, place of birth, residence, or marital or financial status. Sometimes an inability to negotiate these complicated bureaucratic requirements can push the dependent, marginally functioning older person over the brink into the total dependency of an institution.

Family members should help with the bureaucracy, shepherding a mentally impaired old person through the maze of forms and personal interviews, certifications and re-certifications. They must help them to accept these new assistance programs as something to which they are entitled, since these programs are society's response to the skyrocketing costs of health care and the inflationary cost of living, which is hardest on those living on fixed incomes. If the mental impairment of the old relative does not permit him to understand the procedures of application and he is reluctant to sign forms, these agencies will often accept the signature of the next of kin.

Although these procedures may be time-consuming and may occasionally seem demeaning, it is very important to pursue every means of obtaining help. Only in this way can you be sure that all options are available for providing the type of care most appropriate for your relative.

In some instances there are adequate funds for care, but they are in the name of the impaired old person, who refuses to pay. Even before someone becomes mentally impaired, it is generally prudent for families to be aware of the need for joint accounts or trust accounts, or to obtain power of attorney to be able to take care of financial obligations in the event of illness. But if the old person is mistrustful or secretive about his funds, there can be additional problems for the family.

If your relative's mistrustful behavior interferes with your ability to pay his bills or provide care for him, discuss it with his doctor. The physician might prescribe something that will ease your relative's anxieties about his financial affairs and permit him to allow you to help him. If this is not practical, you may have to consult an attorney.

If your kin is accusative and uncooperative, it can be very upsetting. Be sure to include all available family members in trying to work out any problems. Sometimes an impaired relative will trust some members of the family and not others, or he may not be able to hold out against the united opinion of the rest of the family. If this approach also fails, you may find that your relative will give power of attorney to a bank official or a friend.

The important issue is to recognize that you will feel hurt by your relative's behavior if you are not trusted, especially if someone else *is* trusted. You can't help feeling hurt, but if you are prepared for this response, you can overcome it.

These are but a few examples of how financial considerations affect the family's ability to provide care in the
community, and touch upon how it might influence a decision about institutionalization as an option. A dear member of my family used to say, "People are funny about sex
and money!" Isn't it true? We can be totally inconsistent
about money, penny-pinching in some areas and extravagant in others, or we can be consistently frugal or consistently extravagant. Money stands for more than what it
can buy, representing independence, status, and power.
No wonder it can complicate the decision-making process
when assessing the total needs of the impaired older person and his family. It should be confronted as honestly as
possible, so that the meaning of the cost of care and possible loss of income of the impaired member of the family is
balanced against the kind of care he needs and the ability
of his family to provide it.

THE ENVIRONMENT

Sometimes the decisive factor in how long a family keeps a
mentally impaired older person in the community is the
kind of home or neighborhood he lives in. Whether a
home is large enough to have a paid helper sleep in can
make the difference between comfortable management or
a nerve-shattering existence. When the older person needs
twenty four-hour supervision, the family can sometimes
manage with just an aide living in, but that can mean loss
of privacy; because of the high cost of housing, it is generally not feasible to move to larger quarters. But if the older
person lives in an area close to several family members
who can make themselves available to help, this can be the

best arrangement. The family must look to all generations as sources of help.

If the older person lives in his own house or in a spacious apartment, there are more options for his care. And if the older person lives in an area with friendly neighbors, this can be a very significant support in maintaining him in the community. Good neighbors often are helpful, particularly in keeping a watchful eye open or in staying with the impaired older person while the relative or paid helper goes shopping. Whether there is a porch or garden for the older person to sit in, or a safe area for exercise, can also make a big difference in caring for the older person in need of constant supervision. If the community offers a suitable day-care or meals program, that can also help the family to maintain their kin at home.

THE OBSTACLES

Most discussions reflect the attitude that institutionalization should never be the option of choice; it should be turned to only when all other efforts have failed. This attitude persists despite evidence that some alert elderly people enter nursing homes because they believe that a home can meet their physical and social needs better than can the community, where they often feel isolated and lonely. It persists in spite of experience demonstrating that care of the mentally impaired aged can be better in a nursing home than in the community. The attitude is related to the prevailing negative image about the position of the aged in the family and the false view that families dump their elderly into nursing homes and abandon them. In answer to this, some experts point out that families do everything possible to help their elderly and revert to nursing homes only as a last resort, but notice the use of the word *revert*. The word choice itself reveals a bias.

These biases against institutional care are not in the best interests of the mentally impaired aged and their families. At times, such attitudes reflect a genuine and realistic concern for deplorable conditions in many nursing homes or for the excessively high cost of nursing-home care. But although this concern is shared by the public and professionals alike, it is misdirected when it ignores the reality that nursing homes are a vital necessity in the spectrum of services required by the impaired elderly.

In fact, when mental impairment is advanced, the nursing home can offer much better care than the family, unless they have very unusual resources or very substantial finances. The average older family has neither the finances nor the numerous members that would be needed to match the skilled services of the nursing home that are required by the severely impaired aged. But the weight of public opinion against placement in a nursing home, except for the obviously physically impaired, is so strong that most families tend to avoid it until some crisis occurs or is imminent.

APPLICATION

If the family does decide to place its mentally impaired kin in a nursing home, there are other obstacles, which can sometimes seem insurmountable. Finding a suitable nursing home that has a vacancy for the level of care your kin requires and that meets your financial requirements can be an arduous process. Guides to choosing a nursing home list many criteria to watch out for, and experts in long-term care usually advise families to plan ahead and to involve their elderly relatives in selecting a facility. But from years of experience I can tell you that when it comes to the mentally impaired aged, the most decisive factor in placement is often availability and convenience.

How do you determine which is the most suitable facility? First you must know how the care is to be financed. Many nursing homes will not accept Medicaid patients, and some nursing homes will apply for Medicaid only after the patient has been paying the private rate for a specified period—sometimes a few months, sometimes over a year. Other private nursing homes are firm in their policy of nonacceptance of Medicaid and will transfer patients to Medicaid facilities when they or their families are no longer able to pay. The reason behind this is that in many states Medicaid pays a much lower rate than private rates, and the proprietors say that they cannot provide services at those low rates.

Legally, whatever funds are paid by the family for care must be credited toward the Medicaid rate, but you should be aware that in many regions families are told that they can have their relative admitted with Medicaid payments if they agree to pay a supplementary amount. Although this policy is illegal, regulatory agencies sometimes look the other way, since they know that the Medicaid rates in some states are unrealistic. This is a critical social problem, and it results in unequal treatment and sometimes illegal burdens on families from some states.

In general, nonprofit facilities enjoy the best reputation, and usually their admission policies do not discriminate between private paying patients and Medicaid patients. However, they often have long waiting lists, and there may also be an informal practice in some facilities of preferential admissions to people who make donations to the home.

How can you find out about the financial policies and the reputations of nursing homes in your area? If your kin is known to a hospital, ask their social service department for help. If not, you will have to check for yourself to see which is most helpful. Look for the information and referral service of any of the following agencies: local government office for the aging; Community Chest; United Way; Catholic Charities; Federation of Jewish Philanthropies; mental health associations. Sometimes the phone book listing starts with the name of your city. Often the staff of a local senior citizen center is helpful in sharing information about community resources.

You may have to use some ingenuity in finding the information and referral service that is most knowledgeable about nursing homes in terms of financial policy. And you will certainly have to do a lot of telephoning or investigating on your own to find out what the informal policies and vacancy rates are.

The next crucial criterion in the application process is the level of care required by your kin. Before Medicare and Medicaid came about, old people needing institutional care went to homes for the aged (also called rest homes), nursing homes, convalescent homes, or mental hospitals if they were mentally impaired. With Medicare and Medicaid came unanticipated increases in the costs of medical and long-term care, and one result was that regulatory agencies became very concerned about the amount of care that was being given for these very high rates. This led to the development of guidelines and rating scales that document the kind and amount of care that is needed.

Facilities are categorized as *skilled nursing facilities* (SNFs), *intermediate care facilities* (ICFs), and *adult domiciliary care facilities* (ADCFs). In some states the last are called *adult congregate living facilities* (ACLFs).

Basically, an SNF provides total care to someone who needs twenty-four-hour nursing supervision for medical problems. An ICF is for people who need intermittent nursing supervision for what are considered custodial problems. ADCFs provide room and board and help with dressing and bathing, if necessary, and supervision of medications. Many ADCFs are senior residences or hotels that offer these additional services but receive such low rates that the services are often inadequate.

Forms and rating scales have been developed that assess the level of care needed by residents of these facilities according to how they function both physically and mentally. Points are assigned to different categories of needs, such as the need for help with medications, or with dressing, bathing, and toileting. The resident then qualifies for a particular category of care according to the total number of points.

This rating system is not very useful; in fact, it is downright prejudicial to the mentally impaired. It may be obvious that the impaired person needs constant supervision and special care, but these services are not readily quantifiable on a form if they are interpreted literally. However, those working with this process know that the forms can be filled out to show any level of care that you want, and just a little sophistication is needed by the institutional staff to document that level of care in the patients' records. This is an area of frustration for administrators, nurses, doctors, and social workers, who would like simpler, more straightforward assessments, but who are forced into a game-playing attitude by a system obsessed with cost but uncaring or naïve about controlling quality of care.

What all of this means is that a relative of a mentally impaired older person may have to do some digging to learn how the level of care is determined by the institutions he is interested in. It can be particularly difficult to assess the level of care needed by someone with mental impairment, furthermore, because some facilities will say they can be cared for only in their skilled nursing facilities, while the review organization that approves the level of care may insist that they need only custodial care in an intermediate care facility or adult domiciliary care facility. A critical element in this determination is the amount of nursing supervision deemed necessary. If mental impairment can be accepted as a medical condition, it is not unreasonable to point out the need for a nurse to review the patient's medical status regularly.

Before applying for a particular level of care in a specific institution, call and ask for information. Ask what your relative must need in the way of nursing and medical supervision in order to qualify for the different levels of care, and find out what the vacancy rate is for each level. Some nursing homes keep the mentally impaired in specific areas or on certain floors, and they may further separate them according to whether they are able to walk without assistance or whether they are incontinent. They may even be separated according to their level of mental impairment and whether they are agitated and restless, thus requiring more supervision.

Many families cannot accept the necessity for segregating the mentally impaired on separate floors. They often don't consider their kin as deteriorated as a professional assessment describes, and they fear that their relative will deteriorate faster if exposed only to other patients with mental impairment.

There is, however, no evidence that mental decline proceeds faster when the impaired older person is cared for among others of similar mental status. In fact, placing the mentally impaired with alert old people is often less desirable. The alert patient is usually disturbed and frightened, or at least irritated, by the behavior of the confused or disoriented patient, and may shun or even insult him. Those nursing homes that do not separate the mentally impaired from the alert usually make this decision because to them it's more important to fill beds and collect maximum income than to individualize care for patients. Though you may find an environment containing only confused and disturbed patients upsetting at first, keep in mind that the atmosphere is usually more depressing to the family than to the mentally impaired older patient.

Whether a bed is available for your relative will depend upon where he is to be placed, according to the nursing home's criteria. Usually this is more information than can be gotten by telephone, so you will have to be prepared to make appointments for interviews with the people responsible for admissions in the institutions that seem suitable.

The next obstacle for you in the process of placement is the institution's policy about interviewing applicants in person, and its medical examination policies. These policies, which are good practice in dealing with the mentally alert older person, sometimes present overwhelming obstacles for the families of the mentally impaired. If your relative refuses even to visit the nursing home, what can you do? If he is a danger to himself or others, he can be committed for treatment with certification by two doctors, but only to a hospital, not to a nursing home. If you are appointed by the court to become the guardian of his person, you could arrange for nursing-home admission, even against his wishes, but this procedure is traumatic and humiliating. Because of very narrow definitions of competency, it is even difficult to have someone declared incompetent. For example, a psychiatrist sent by the Protective Services Division of the Department of Human Services to an old woman whose neighbors complained that she was a danger because she set fires, stated that he could not declare her incompetent because she knew her name and address. He would not violate her civil rights if she was "only senile."

With such confusion among professionals as to what constitutes mental competency and the ability to function in the community, it is easy to see why families may find themselves in a state of total desperation when trying to place a mentally impaired older person who cannot recognize his need for care and protection.

Many nursing homes require only a medical report that can be filled out by the private physician, but some require a personal interview and a medical examination by the staff of the institution. If your relative is nervous about the interview or the exam, your private doctor may order some medication to reduce his anxieties. Sometimes the institution will modify its procedures to accommodate the mentally impaired applicant by scheduling the personal interview and medical exam on the same day. Be sure to ask if this is possible, since each time you have to bring your kin to the institution may be traumatic for all involved.

Another important consideration in placement is the

location of the facility. If the institution does not have its own medical staff, you may want to arrange for placement in a facility that is convenient for the patient's private doctor. If that is not an important issue for you, then you will want to find the best possible facility that is convenient for family visiting.

What if your kin lives in another state? Is it better to try to arrange placement where he lives, or move him near you so that you can visit and supervise his care? This can be a very difficult question to answer. Generally it is considered good practice to maintain as consistent an environment as possible. If your kin lives in a very different climate, it may be difficult for him to adjust to the change. On the other hand, when the change is a move to an institution, he may not notice the change in climate. A more serious obstacle may be the governing residency requirements for Medicaid eligibility if your kin does not have sufficient funds to be a private paying resident for at least one year.

According to a United States Supreme Court ruling on eligibility for welfare, it is illegal for any state to disqualify someone for Medicaid based on a requirement for residency in the state, but some states are in fact turning down applications on the basis of residency. The excuse used by the state to disqualify someone who has moved there for the purpose of receiving nursing-home care is that the regulations prohibit anyone from entering a state for the sole purpose of becoming a recipient of medical services. But since it can be shown that medical services are available in every state, and the family of the impaired older person is residing in the state to which he wants to move, it can be demonstrated that the reason for the move is not to receive medical services but to be close to the family. When the families involved demand a fair hearing from the Medicaid office, these decisions can be overruled, but most institutions are unwilling to admit patients knowing in advance that they may have to wait a long time for payment until the case is heard. All in all, it may prove too difficult to arrange nursing-home admission from one state to another.

What if your kin cannot be managed in the community any longer, and there is no suitable vacancy in the nursing home of your choice? Should you move your relative into a less desirable facility until a vacancy becomes available in the preferred nursing home? Is it possible to arrange for a transfer in the future? Once again, this can prove to be a difficult problem. While a transfer is theoretically possible, there are many obstacles. First, you may find it impossible to locate a nursing home that is willing to admit a confused older person if the institution knows in advance that the admission is temporary. It is more prudent to arrange the placement without revealing your hope for future transfer. In fact, you may find that after your relative adjusts to his new home, you will not want to upset his routines by transferring him to a new environment. Furthermore, if the preferred nursing home is more desirable because of its better reputation and facilities, there is probably so much demand for vacancies that priority will not be given to someone already placed in a nursing home.

One last point concerning why it may be difficult to place your kin in the facility that has the best reputation. Most such facilities have several levels of care. As residents in the intermediate levels become more impaired and require more skilled care, they are transferred to the areas more heavily staffed for the increased services. So, as vacancies occur, they are more often for people requiring a lower level of care. Since families often wait to place

THE PARADOX OF INSTITUTIONAL CARE 203

mentally impaired relatives until they may need a heavy level of care, they are not likely to find vacancies of that level in the facilities of their choice.

Be aware that the finest facilities have a limited number of beds and cannot possibly admit everyone who would like to come there. Be prepared to accept the best available vacancy, even though it may not be your first choice. Be aware too that even the best facilities fall short of ideal in the everyday provision of care.

What if all these obstacles are overcome—your doctor has been cooperative in getting your relative through the application process, a vacancy is available—and then your relative refuses to go? Don't despair. It usually works out, although not necessarily as planned. Sometimes the older person is cooperative up until the moment of admission, and then says, "Oh, no. You're not getting me in there!" Or, in answer to your explanations and reasonings, he says, "If the home is so great, *you* go there!"

If you discuss this problem with the staff of the nursing home, they will suggest techniques for getting your relative to try out the facility. Your anxiety about the move will be felt by your relative, so it's important to get as much help as possible from others in the family and from the staff of the nursing home. Most experts will advise honesty in handling the move and suggest changing the subject when your relative gets upset. Be sure to get some medication from the doctor to lessen your kin's fears, and try to be matter-of-fact in spite of your strong emotions. Arranging for nursing-home admission for your kin, after determining that it is the best plan, calls for "courage to change what should be changed."

I have tried in this chapter to show the many factors influencing the decision of some families to place their severely impaired kin in institutions, while other families elect to allow their similarly impaired relatives to remain in the community. Sometimes the mentally impaired older person is treated more poorly at home than he would be in a nursing home. An overwrought, angry care-giver may use sarcasm and insults when dealing with difficult behavior. The impaired older person may or may not be aware of it, but the situation is certainly less than satisfactory. Or the exhausted family may be verging on collapse, while the well-cared-for older person is oblivious of his surroundings, unaware of who it is who cares for him.

The paradox is that even when the institution clearly would provide better care, it is viewed as less desirable than family care. It is my hope that as families learn more about mental impairment, they will also learn under which circumstances the institution can offer better care. And when they are accepted by the institution as members of a caring team, the result can be the best possible treatment for one of the worst possible conditions. The responsible family must recognize and sort through its complex emotions and practical problems. Only then can it start to overcome the burden of negative public opinion about institutionalization and place in proper perspective the needs of the entire family, including the mentally impaired older person. In time, the public will learn that under certain circumstances the decision to institutionalize can be the most reasonable—and humane—of all options.

11

Coping with the Institution

*L*et's start this difficult chapter with a cheerful story. Mrs. Chase's family was troubled for months about the necessity of placing her in a nursing home. They had been supplying round-the-clock help for her, but they couldn't afford it indefinitely. Finally they arranged for her admission to the best nursing home that would admit someone of her severe level of confusion. They were upset, fearing that she would not adjust to sharing a room and that she would be disturbed to be in such a depressing environment.

The day after Mrs. Chase's admission, the social

worker visited her to see how she was getting along and to determine what might help in her adjustment. "How are you, Mrs. Chase? How do you like your new home?" she asked pleasantly. Mrs. Chase smiled with surprise. "New home? Why, my dear, I've been coming to this church all my life!"

What Mrs. Chase's family dreaded never came to pass. She had no trouble adjusting, because her level of confusion was such that the new environment made her feel that she was in her church. The nurse and aides all addressed her by name, and she felt comfortable with so many friendly folks around.

Very often the mentally impaired older person makes a much easier adjustment than do his anxious relatives, who sometimes act as though they are consigning him to a funeral home rather than a nursing home.

Where do these deeply felt emotions come from? What do you have to know to overcome them?

THE ASYLUM COMPLEX

Many people have no experience with nursing homes or other institutions until they need to find one for an aging impaired relative. In fact, as recently as 1939 there were only 1,200 nursing homes in this country; by 1975, there were 25,000.

In former times, when very few people survived to really old age, there were usually enough family members available to provide care for the infirm. Those needing help who had no families and were poor would end up in the poorhouse or almshouse, public infirmary, mental hospital, or other kind of asylum. The patients were called "inmates," just as though they were in jail, and there were very negative attitudes attached to the institutions. People had good reason to dread these places, because inmates were treated as pariahs, stripped of individual identity and dignity. Conditions were deplorable, particularly because so little public money was allocated for the sick and insane.

Although our social structure has since changed, and nursing homes serve a totally different clientele, these very negative attitudes persist. Placing a relative in a nursing home is experienced as a social stigma requiring explanations to anyone who will listen. No matter how obvious it is that the relative who is being placed for care is severely impaired and beyond the capability of the family, those involved in placement usually feel uncomfortable and guilty. I call this reaction an "asylum complex."

The members of the staff in most nursing homes recognize the extreme pain the family feels during the process of placement, and usually they try to help them. Wanting to be reassuring, they say things like "Don't worry. Your mother's in good hands now. We know how to take care of her. We will help her to get used to her new home. Just leave it all to us." You can see how such reassurances would add to feelings of family failure.

But although the staff tries to be helpful in the beginning, the honeymoon is often over as soon as the family raises the first questions about the care being given to the new resident in the nursing home. The family members frequently feel that the staff adds to their guilt and makes them feel powerless in the face of what they perceive as inadequate care. How does this happen? Why is it such a common lament? An understanding of the nursing home as a system can help clarify the issues.

THE SYSTEM

Nursing homes vary according to size, location, sponsorship, and source of funds. Most of them are privately owned and operated and not larger than 100 beds. Some are public institutions, and still others are private, nonprofit homes established by religious or charitable organizations or fraternal orders.

Since the arrival of Medicare and Medicaid, government funds have become a primary source of payment for nursing-home care, leading to an unanticipated degree of government influence on the health-care system. Federal and state agencies have established regulations and standards for nursing-home care, and these have had a profound impact on the whole system. While basic services improved in many institutions, costs skyrocketed, resulting in stricter criteria as to eligibility for care. This in turn led to ridiculous quantities of paperwork, which left less time for direct care of nursing-home residents.

The nursing home is an organization whose purpose is to provide a specified level of personal and health care to a specific clientele. To provide this care, there is a staff consisting of an administrator, nurses, aides, housekeeping help, dietary workers, clerks, and secretaries. Depending upon the size of the home, there are physicians, therapists, pharmacists, activity workers, and social workers, either part-time or full-time.

Where there are many different kinds of personnel of varying skills and experience, there must be a hierarchy of authority, with established rules and regulations. Favoritism must be avoided toward staff and patients. Strict adherence to rules and regulations, however, can cause difficulties in meeting the individual needs of patients and their families, and the requirement for a "chain of command" can create conflicts among the staff of the organization.

In a nursing home the ideal method of meeting the complex needs of the individual patient is the "team approach," in which all staff members involved in providing care share their special knowledge of the patient to formulate a coordinated plan of care. The members of the team, however, are not always successful in suspending professional biases when there are differences in opinion, and they may have trouble agreeing on a treatment plan that balances medical and nursing needs with social and psychological factors. Furthermore, the observations and opinions of the aides, who usually feel they know the patient best, are often overlooked or unsolicited. Remember, to paraphrase George Orwell, although everyone in a democracy is supposed to be equal, some are more equal than others.

How personnel are treated in an organization obviously affects morale, and the morale of the staff is part of what can be called the "climate" of an organization. Be aware that the climate can vary from one section of the institution to another, from one floor to another, and from one shift to another. The kind of care that is provided is very much influenced by the institutional climate and satisfaction (or lack of it) of the staff.

Very often what is perceived by the family as unfeeling or brusque behavior by the personnel of the nursing home may reflect dissatisfaction among the staff. And criticizing areas of neglect by a conscientious nursing staff overwhelmed with paperwork can add to their frustration and bring forth a defensive or angry response. The family member who is upset by the need for placement to begin with, and further upset at having to mention problems, is usually devastated by the staff's angry responses. It is crucial to recognize that the underlying cause of the anger is not necessarily the relative making the complaint, but the system.

Whether or not a nursing home is unionized also has a significant effect on the system. As in many organizations, employees may have voted to be represented by a union in labor matters. In some ways the union has a positive effect on the system if employee morale improves, but since the primary goal of the union is the protection of its employees, at times it can hinder good care if there is a conflict between patients' and employees' needs.

The patient's family is also part of the nursing-home system, although most homes do not provide a formal role for them. If administrators of nursing homes could only appreciate the potential usefulness of the family as part of the system, they would try to develop some sort of formal function—such as family councils, which could provide a mechanism for the family to learn more about the nursing home, to talk to other families, and to carve out meaningful roles for themselves. Unfortunately, however, family councils are sometimes viewed as "gripe sessions," or opportunities for complaining, and administrators are generally opposed to them.

Perhaps the most significant element in appreciating the complexity of the nursing home as a system is the effect of the personality, values, and personal attributes of each member of the staff system and how he thinks he is being treated by the patients and their families. For example, personal attributes that will probably affect the interaction among family members and staff are social status of the staff members, their intelligence and experience level, and their feelings about their own families. Their personal values will determine how they judge the behavior and requests of the families of patients.

Most of the aides in nursing homes come from disadvantaged groups who traditionally have a strong sense of family solidarity and interdependence and feel that members of the family should be cared for at home. They would not place an elderly relative in an institution except under extreme circumstances. They are often unaware that this strong personal value is reflected in a judgmental attitude toward the relatives who leave their aged kin in their care. They may well treat the patients as though they are their own family, but they tend to be antagonistic to and intolerant of the real family if they feel it is interfering.

Personal attributes influence interaction with staff at professional levels as well. One never knows whether brusque handling by the charge nurse is due to poor timing of a request, or to a migraine headache caused by her teenage children.

The nursing home is not an isolated system, but is affected by all other elements in society, such as the political climate, the state of competition among agencies for funds, the availability of skilled staff. The degree of vigilance by governmental regulatory agencies will also affect the dynamics of the system, as well as the presence of volunteers and visitors in the institution.

This extremely complex view of the nursing home as a system composed of subsystems, operating within the larger social system, should provide a background for better understanding the problems we will discuss, which are commonly expressed by families of patients.

When your relative is admitted to a nursing home or similar institution for long-term care, you go through one of life's final transitions, and like all transitions, this one engenders mixed emotions. The first day you send your child to school is filled with apprehension and joy, and so are other rites of passage—confirmations, graduations, engagements and marriages, new jobs, promotions. Life also challenges us with crises that bring fear and unhappiness—loss of employment, divorce, bereavement, chronic illness, and disability. If we are able to channel the emotional energy that the crisis generates into some positive action, then the experience can create an opportunity for growth.

ADMISSION TASKS

The first tasks facing you upon placing your impaired kin in an institution are practical ones. What suggestions does the nursing home make as to clothing? Do they have a system for marking items with a laundry pen so that they won't get lost, or do you have to buy name labels and sew them in? How often is clothing laundered and how many changes are needed? How much closet and drawer space is there?

One of the deepest feelings of anguish occurs when you must put all your relative's possessions into one small closet and two or three drawers! It *has* to be experienced as a stripping away of part of the identity of your relative as a person. It *is* sad, and you may cry. But then you must accept this as a practical necessity.

If possible, try to involve your kin in the choices as to which clothing and personal possessions to take, and what to do with the possessions that remain. If you can store some of the items yourself, you don't have to make all of these decisions at one time, and you can replenish the wardrobe with familiar clothing when it is needed.

You will also need to put all valuables away for safe-keeping. Jewelry must be removed, since there is an obvious danger of loss or theft. Despite the confusion of the old person, many families are reluctant to remove such valuables as diamond keepsake rings. But once the older person is scheduled for admission to a nursing home, the family must be practical about removing rings, valuable watches, and similar heirlooms. These belongings frequently disappear immediately after admission, since it is really difficult for the institution to keep track of them unless they are checked into a business office safe.

The same holds true for cash. A minimum of spending money, if any, should be left with the mentally impaired older person. This often is a source of stress, since the older person may be used to having some cash in his pocket at all times. He may continually ask for money, saying he won't be able to get anything to eat. The staff should be skilled in managing such anxious patients. You may find that your relative is reassured by a note from you stating that his money is in the bank for safekeeping or that you are holding it for him. Discuss ways of handling this with the staff, if it seems to be a problem, but don't fall into the trap of leaving cash with your relative with the feeling that you don't mind if it's lost or stolen. It *will* be lost or stolen, and your relative will have even more reason for worrying that he has no money.

Try to make your relative's room as cozy as possible, within the regulations established by the nursing home. Some pictures on the dresser and wall, a few bright pillows, a favorite throw, and some plants can make a big difference. If your relative's mental condition is such that he is no longer aware of his surroundings or cannot express his feelings about his placement, don't feel that your efforts are useless. At some point or on some level, your relative may be aware of his environment.

Some nursing homes may have rules against bringing in plants or other items that need special attention. They may not want to take responsibility for cleaning a personal blanket or pillow. They may disclaim responsibility for possessions, fearing they might be stolen. They may feel that watering plants and cleaning up spills are excessive work for the housekeeping staff. If you offer to have the blanket cleaned yourself or to assume the risk of theft or to water the plants, you may find the nursing-home administrator more supportive.

However, if you run into a rigid policy, an administration that says, "If I make an exception to this rule, everyone will want plants and pillows," don't be disheartened. Give it time. You can't change rigid policies all at once, but you can try a series of compromises. Start with whatever seems most important to you. Ask to speak with the person in charge at a convenient time. Let him know that you understand how difficult his job must be—complying with regulations, managing budgets, handling staff, and arranging for the care of so many helpless patients. But ask if he would consider allowing you to make your relative's room more homelike with one plant or one pillow or one blanket. Say you'll take responsibility for it and that you'll remove it if it causes problems. They say you can catch more flies with honey than with vinegar, and it's usually worth a try. But if you are not sincere in expressing a genuine understanding of the problems of a large organization, you may find that your suggested compromises are viewed as a technique to challenge authority and therefore are resisted by management. If, after a reasonable period of time, you still feel it is an important issue, try again.

Be sure that you've identified the person in charge of the decision you are looking for. Sometimes a family member is told by the aide or a nurse that he can't do something for the patient—it's a policy or a rule. Often the family member simply accepts the so-called rule unquestioningly, building up resentment if it is obviously unfair, without trying to learn who sets the rules and who can change them. Learn the chain of command. (See Appendix 5.) Don't be timid about asking for relaxation of rules. But do it with consideration for the total operation of the institution.

THE STAFF

On the day of your relative's admission, find out who will be responsible for his care. It is important to know which nurses, aides, and orderlies will be primarily responsible. Sometimes family members are so upset by the admission procedures—which may involve signing contracts, turning over bankbooks or insurance papers, and so on—that they forget the amenities. Be sure to introduce yourself and greet as many of the staff as possible. If you can overcome your anxieties enough to be friendly to all the staff, it will be a better beginning for your new relationships. Each time you visit, make it your business to look around for the staff to greet them. If you can take some time to get to know a little about each member, it will result in better care for your relative.

To accept you as a partner in caring for your kin, the staff in the institution must take you into the partnership.

They must see you as *involved* but not *interfering*. This depends not only on your tact and understanding and timing in raising concerns about your relative, but on the tact and understanding of the staff member with whom you are speaking. No matter how sensitively you remind the staff of something that needs doing, you risk its being interpreted as a criticism, and few people like criticism.

Very often the family is reluctant to ask the staff to take care of some need of their relative, because they feel guilty that the staff is doing the dirty work they couldn't manage. They may feel that being an aide or attendant is such a low-status and low-paying occupation that they shouldn't add to the burden by asking for a service, even when it is necessary.

The occupation of aide or attendant is as worthy as any other honest job, and it's not really more difficult than many others. Emptying a bedpan may be viewed by some as undesirable work, but is it more unpleasant than a rectal examination done by a physician? The issue is not the dirty work itself, but the attitude of those who perform it. Many aides take pride in their work, particularly when they are part of an institution that gives them recognition for good performance. Many aides prefer their jobs to other occupations they might find boring and uninteresting, such as factory work.

So don't wallow in misplaced guilt, feeling that the aides must resent you for expecting them to be proficient in tasks that you couldn't do. Even if it makes you feel uncomfortable, there are times when you must be direct in pointing out something your relative needs for his safety or comfort.

Some experts have advised relatives not to be afraid to speak up. They say complaints do not bring retaliation;

instead they make problems more visible and lead to solutions. Well, it doesn't always work that way. A favorite trump card used by staff members who feel harassed by a particular relative is to say, "I'm sorry that we're not able to give your mother the kind of care you'd like. If you're so dissatisfied, why don't you take her home?"

What a low blow! It's a calculated cruelty, since nursing-home staffs well know that families place their kin in nursing homes only when they can't be managed any longer in the community. A similar response, although not as sadistic as the previous one, is by the nurse or aide who says, "Your mother has that problem only when you're here. When you're not around, she's fine." That's the staff's way of getting back at you by playing on your asylum complex. It's sure to make you feel powerless.

Prepare yourself for these responses. Recognize that the staff has feelings too. Voice your concern only about serious problems. And then try not to be intimidated by a staff that may be irritable from tedious and sometimes unpleasant work with sometimes difficult patients. After all, if the difficult patients were removed, their services would be unnecessary!

THE TREATMENT PLAN

On the day of admission, let the nurse in charge know that you would like to be informed of your relative's treatment plan. Usually the family is asked to bring all medications that the patient has been taking, but these medications are not necessarily continued. The physician in charge of your kin's care in the nursing home is supposed to do a complete physical examination shortly after admission, and he will write new orders for medications and other therapies. The family should take an active role in knowing what medication their relative is taking, what it is for, and what effect it should have. Medications are often dropped or added when a patient is admitted, and although it is the responsibility of the nursing staff to observe the patient from that time on, the family should feel free to discuss any changes in appearance or behavior of which they become aware. This is especially important in the beginning, since the family still knows the patient better than the staff does.

Even when the patient is admitted to a nursing home directly from a hospital, and written medical orders are sent along, it is prudent for the family to inquire about the treatment plan and medications. Sometimes orders are written so illegibly that mistakes are made. The interest of the family can remind the staff to be thorough in understanding transfer documents and other medical records.

Be sure to check on whether your relative has been used to taking particular laxatives and whether his treatment plan includes them. If there is a change of routine ordered, follow up with the nurse in a few days as to whether your relative is eliminating normally. Since he is mentally impaired, he cannot be expected to be responsible for himself, even in this highly personal area. If problems develop with constipation, they may be overlooked at the beginning, and since those problems can cause other problems, constipation is a legitimate area for concern.

Once your relative has settled in, your involvement in his treatment and medication has to change. You must assume that the staff is doing its job properly, unless there is evidence to the contrary. You cannot expect to discuss your relative's condition every time you visit. There aren't enough personnel to do that. But if you notice changes in his condition, then it *is* appropriate to discuss this with the nurse in charge.

It is one function of the social worker to get to know everything relevant about your relative so that his social and psychological needs will be met as far as possible. For example, his former interests and skills should be noted so that activities with the recreation worker or occupational therapist can be arranged. However, many institutions do not provide an adequate number of social workers. If no social worker is available, talk to the nurse in charge about your relative's background and ask if you can talk to the recreation worker. Perhaps you can share some important clues as to what may still interest your relative.

It is also very important to let the staff know about any food preferences or habits. Although it is impossible to meet every individual taste, where there are choices available, the staff will probably try to accommodate. Family members can meet an important need by taking special food treats when they visit. This serves the dual purpose of making visits more enjoyable and sharing in an area of care that is beyond the capability of an institution. For example, ethnic foods are generally not part of nursing-home dietary repertoires, except perhaps on special occasions. Since food is often symbolic of giving and loving, the family is able to show loving feelings by bringing special foods. Two cautions, however: be sure to check with the nursing staff about whether there are any restrictions in your kin's diet, and take care not to cause any sanitary problems by leaving food behind in improper containers.

How a resident accepts having a roommate is another unpredictable issue to be faced upon admission. It is important to introduce the roommates by name, although they probably will not remember them. Sometimes roommates feel compatible; other times they feel like intruders. Don't overreact if the first few encounters are not friendly. Let the staff handle it. This is part of their expertise.

When you leave your relative alone in the nursing home, you may feel relieved or devastated. After that, there will be times when you will feel frustrated, regretful, angry with the staff, hurt, and powerless. And there will be good times, when you realize that your kin is getting the care he needs. Remind yourself always that the basic problems you may experience are not caused by your inadequacies or the institution's, but by the condition that is responsible for your relative's level of mental impairment.

COMMON COMPLAINTS

Most problems that arise for families and staff are related generally to patients' clothing and personal appearance and to the specific problems of missing false teeth and eyeglasses.

Clothing

No matter how carefully the family has marked the patient's clothing, or how good a system the nursing home has for collecting, cleaning, and returning it, clothing seems to get lost. Sometimes it is returned to the wrong floor, sometimes to the wrong room on the right floor. Sometimes it's in the wrong closet in the right room. Sometimes a confused resident wanders into someone else's room and puts on his clothing. Sometimes a resident doesn't have enough items of clothing for sufficient changes between laundering, and an aide borrows clothing from another resident.

Whatever the reason for the missing clothing, it is a source of irritation for the relatives. Too often, staff plays on the guilt of the relatives, making them feel it's impossible to keep track of so many items of clothing, having as a ready-made excuse the confusion of the residents. It's more a matter of good organization and good supervision than anything else. The frequent assumption that someone on staff stole the clothing is usually false, as is the staff's assertion that another resident took it. A thorough investigation usually turns up the missing items eventually.

It is understandable that relatives are upset when they visit and find their kin dressed in strange clothing. Since the clothing we wear becomes part of our identity, finding a confused relative dressed in somebody else's clothes is experienced as another level of stripping away of the person's identity. Some upset relatives simply give up on the institution and keep buying clothing replacements. Some take the clothing home to launder themselves, even though the rates charged by the nursing home generally include a normal amount of laundering.

There is a commonsense approach to this problem. First, check on whether your kin has enough changes of clothing to last from laundry pickup to delivery, taking into consideration holidays and other days off. This is determined by whether your kin is incontinent and whether he is able to stay clean or makes a mess at meals. Discuss with the staff in charge whether there is adequate, appropriate clothing for his condition, or whether his clothing still fits him. If, after such a discussion, you've made sure there is enough clothing and it still disappears, try to find out from the staff in charge (usually the floor nurse) what

CARING FOR THE MENTALLY IMPAIRED ELDERLY

the problem is. If the explanation is unreasonable and seems more like an excuse, discuss the problem with a person at a higher level of authority, either a nursing supervisor or an administrator. If you demonstrate that you understand the complexities of the situation, you should get some action from the institution. But if you don't get satisfaction, try not to feel too defeated by the system. Ask yourself how important it is and whether it's worth the energy to battle it through, then act accordingly.

Grooming

Sometimes family members are upset by changes in their kin's appearance. They may be walking around with stockings knotted above the knees, they may need a shave or haircut, or they may suddenly have a strange hairstyle. Someone who had colored her hair may now have gray hair growing in. A previously fastidious person may now have food all over his clothing. He may stop wearing his dentures or his glasses. Finally, a family member may be startled by an extreme weight gain or weight loss.

How important are these issues, and what can be done about them? The first question to be answered is, for whom is this a problem? If your kin is unaware of the change in his appearance, then it is important only insofar as you or other visitors are upset by the change. Then you must find out how complicated it would be to correct the situation. You must also find out if the change is indicative of potential problems for your kin, in which case you must approach the situation with a greater degree of urgency.

For example, discuss with the staff in charge how you feel about the knotted stockings. Find out if the problem is that your relative is uncooperative in being helped to put on the old stocking supports, or if it takes too long for the staff to manage it. It could be that your kin has become incontinent, and needs many more changes of stockings and support garments than she has. Whatever the reason, if you discuss your feelings about this change in your relative's appearance, perhaps you and the staff can work out a solution together.

If you are upset at finding your relative unshaven, discuss this with the staff in the same way. You might point out that you realize your relative doesn't mind being unshaven, but it bothers you. You might learn that those residents who need assistance with shaving receive that service only twice a week, when a male aide is available or when the barber comes. Or perhaps your relative is used to a type of razor that the staff does not use and therefore makes it very difficult for them to keep him shaved. Or your relative might allow one person on the staff to shave him, but not another. You can work on a solution accordingly. You can supply the familiar razor if the staff will use it, or request that the preferred staff member be assigned more often. You can try to shave him yourself when you visit. Or you can learn to accept the change in appearance, since this is not a matter of basic health and safety.

Why might your relative have a strange new hairstyle? If your kin is taken to a new beautician who does not know how she used to have her hair done, obviously she may come out looking different. If you feel this is important, you should discuss your kin's hairstyle with the staff person in charge before she goes to the beautician. Many nursing homes have the aides wash and comb the residents' hair, and your kin's appearance will be related to how skillful or interested they are. Some relatives are pleasantly surprised at *improvements* in their kin's appearance, thanks to the special skills of the staff. All changes, after all, are not bad! But if your experience is a sad one, discuss your feelings with the staff and see whether you might share in this area, by taking your kin on occasion to her previous beautician or by learning to set her hair yourself during your visits.

Hair color is more of a challenge, because most nursing homes don't have facilities for bleaching or dyeing hair. Unless you take responsibility for taking your relative out for this procedure, you will probably find it more practical to allow the hair to grow in with its natural color. You may find that your relative's level of confusion makes it too difficult to take her to a beauty parlor for such lengthy and complicated procedures. Sometimes a wig can be helpful during the process of letting hair grow back in its natural color, but remember that if your relative's mental impairment is very advanced, she may not be able to understand how to use the wig. Be realistic before going out and buying a costly wig that might not be usable by your relative.

If you are disturbed by messy clothing, remember that accidents can happen at every meal and after meals, and you can't reasonably expect a change of clothing three times a day or more. But you can discuss with the staff whether some kind of smock could be used during meals, keeping in mind that your relative would have to be cooperative about wearing it (this may be troublesome, since it would be an unaccustomed type of garment) and that the institution would have to be willing to take care of the extra laundry.

Dentures

The issue of dentures is complex and challenging, primarily because there are so many reasons to remove them and so many places for them to get lost. I remember one newly admitted resident who removed his dentures during a meal and wrapped them in a paper napkin on his tray. The tray was routinely cleaned and the napkin thrown into the trash and eventually into the garbage compactor. By the time anyone noticed that the resident was missing his dentures, it was too late. The relative knew that it was a habit for the old man to remove his dentures during meals at home, but he did not anticipate the routine of the nursing home, where anything left on a tray in a napkin would go in the garbage.

Once dentures are lost, it may be impossible to have a new set made that will be comfortable enough to guarantee that the mentally impaired older person will use them. Since the person might have difficulty in being fitted properly, usually because he doesn't understand the dentist's instructions or is unable to let the dentist know what is comfortable or not, it is generally not practical to have new dentures made at this stage. Family members are often not able to accept this without trying, so they often insist on having new dentures made, only to find that their kin won't wear them.

The most important thing is to try to prevent losses. All dentures should be marked with some kind of engraving instrument that would identify them if lost. It is not uncommon for confused roommates to wear each other's dentures, even though it may seem impossible to imagine that they wouldn't notice. Sometimes this results in sore gums, removal and misplacement of the offending dentures, and a cycle of inability to eat properly, and loss of weight, and ill-fitting dentures because of weight loss.

The change in appearance of someone who no longer wears dentures or whose dentures are loose and clicking when he talks is one of the most painful changes to which the family must adjust.

Eyeglasses

Equally important is the change in appearance due to lost glasses or to a patient's inability to remember to wear glasses. Glasses are lost so frequently by the forgetful older person that they should be routinely marked in an institution. Confused residents often pick up someone else's glasses and then cannot understand why they can't see properly. Someone who no longer remembers to put on glasses to read obviously will stop reading. In the same way, if a resident needs glasses to watch television, the staff should be instructed to remind him to put on his glasses. This is often overlooked. A patient can lose interest in watching TV, when the picture is blurred. We have no way of knowing what effect this decreased amount of stimulation might be having.

It is important for you to make the staff aware of your concern that your relative's glasses be marked and kept track of and that the staff take responsibility for reminding him to put on his glasses when needed.

Weight Gain or Loss

The final reason for a change in appearance, obvious weight gain or weight loss, once again emphasizes the need for family attentiveness to changes, for communication with the staff. Most such changes will be observed by the nursing staff and discussed as part of a treatment plan, but the family has a right and a responsibility to be aware of the reason for such changes. When someone is gaining weight, it might be related to the person's eating more in the institution than he ate at home, but it could reflect an increase in appetite as a side effect of medication, or a decrease in the amount of exercise. It may be that eating is a substitute for other activities. It could be that the confused older person forgets that he has eaten and gets snacks in a coffee shop, or is eating only sweets or carbohydrates because of changes in how food tastes to him. Or he may be sneaking food from other residents' trays in the dining room. The important thing is for the staff to investigate the cause of the weight gain and do what can be done to correct it if necessary.

More common is weight loss. This can occur as a normal process in aging, or it may reflect a need for more individual attention to finding appealing foods or taking adequate time to encourage eating. Sometimes an old person at a very advanced stage of impairment needs to be fed and this may require so much time that he is not being adequately nourished. This is a challenge for the institution and the family.

There are cases where an older person needs up to an hour to be fed, and it is very difficult for an institution to give that amount of staff time to this activity. Sometimes volunteers are recruited for this purpose. Sometimes family members come to help with feeding under these circumstances, although some institutions discourage this degree of family involvement. Why might this happen? Wouldn't the nursing home be grateful for the family's help?

The only plausible reason for not allowing the family to help with feeding is that it is felt that family members are too critical of the many problems they witness when they spend a great deal of time in the dining room. This points up the need for the institution to educate the family as to its role in the nursing home. By helping families to understand the nature of the problems they may witness, institutions can keep family members from overreacting. Where the institution does not take this responsibility, family members must try to help one another to function effectively within the system, and to demonstrate to the nursing-home staff that they understand their difficulties and are seeking ways to improve conditions together.

NEGLECT

Once your relative has "settled in," you will undoubtedly develop expectations about the quality of care he should get. You have every reason to expect that your kin will be protected, groomed, nourished, adequately treated, and well cared for in general. The reality is that even in the best institutions there will be times when residents wander off, when someone is disheveled, when someone is injured because of inadequate supervision, to mention just a few of the problems that may arise.

In some of the smaller homes, it may be easier to supervise care than it is in a large facility with long corridors and many rooms. For example, you may have placed your relative because he had started to wander out of the house and was in danger of being lost. A large nursing home will have elevators, and the charge nurse cannot keep an eye on them every minute. A confused resident may get into an elevator and wander out of the building. Usually there are enough personnel to prevent this: aides, housekeeping staff, security officers, even switchboard operators or re-

ceptionists perform the surveillance duties needed for confused residents, who are no longer kept in locked wards.
But occasionally a resident slips by when staff members
are occupied with other tasks. Although you would be
rightfully upset if your relative was the rare one to get lost,
you must realize that it is impossible to protect someone
completely. Even when a patient has the luxury of a private nurse or companion, there are moments when the
patient may be left alone (when the nurse is in the bathroom, for instance), at which time the patient may get into
trouble.

This should not be labeled as neglect if it is something
that happens only rarely. No one can reasonably expect
100-percent protection, 100 percent of the time. You can
only expect as much protection as possible under the circumstances. But if one of the main reasons for placing
your relative was his protection, you cannot help but feel
devastated when problems arise that you feel could have
been prevented by closer supervision.

Sometimes accidents occur just because the older person has been moved into a new environment. I have heard
families complain on occasion that if they had known their
relatives would not be completely protected, they would
never have moved them into a nursing home—they might
as well have taken their chances leaving them at home. At
such moments they are forgetting the extent of problems
at home, which might have continued to worsen. It should
be kept in mind that an impaired old person is at risk
wherever he is, and the decision to institutionalize is made
to minimize danger. But danger cannot be eliminated altogether.

When patients are no longer able to walk safely alone,
or when they are no longer ambulatory at all, they are

sometimes kept in restraints or seated in special geriatric chairs with trays that lock to keep the patient from falling out. Although this is done for the patient's protection, the family is often upset by this further evidence of deterioration. If the older person cries to be freed from what he may feel is a state of bondage, it can indeed by devastating to witness.

The family must discuss this with the nursing staff to learn whether the restraints have been ordered by a doctor or whether they are being used because there's not enough staff to keep the older person from wandering or otherwise endangering himself. Questions should be raised as to whether enough effort has been made to provide appropriate activities as distractions. Restraints may be used only on medical orders, and the orders should specify how long they are to be used. This rule is a safeguard against the misuse of restraints. If restraints are clearly necessary for the older person's protection, the family must try to accept them, but if the patient becomes agitated when restrained, the family should also discuss the use of appropriate medication. As always, the physician must find the right dosage of the correct medication for the comfort of the patient, being alert to his changing needs as his condition changes.

Families sometimes plead with the nursing staff to allow the vulnerable older person to stay in bed, which may seem more comfortable or simply more dignified than being restrained in a chair. But they must learn that it is medically necessary for a frail old person to be gotten out of bed regularly to prevent bed sores, lung congestion, and other medical hazards.

Another area of frequent complaint concerns problems related to incontinence and whether patients are changed often enough. This can be a difficult problem for staff to keep up with, but the institution *must* assign sufficient aides to keep patients comfortable and free of bedsores. This does not mean that your relative will be dry every time you visit. It would be impossible to change patients as soon as they wet themselves, but they should not go unchanged for too long.

Too often, if housekeeping is poor and nursing care inadequate, the major objection by visitors to a nursing home can be the smell of incontinence that permeates the entire institution. This is unnecessary and unacceptable. Well-run institutions demonstrate that they can be free of unpleasant odors. There may be temporary odors until staff has had the time to clean up, but a pervasive odor is evidence of lack of proper care, and it should be reported to the ombudsman committee of the local department of health, if discussions with the staff prove to be fruitless. If you have been forced to accept this type of nursing home because nothing else was available, it does not mean there is no hope for improvement. If enough families get together to voice their disapproval, and if the local department of health is informed, the condition can be overcome.

Try to be realistic in your expectations. Don't expect total supervision, but don't settle for too little. How can you know what's too little and what's too much to expect? By using old-fashioned common sense, by recognizing when your emotions may be interfering with your good judgment, and by talking your problems over with responsible staff members and with other relatives who are going through similar difficulties. Always remember and practice the motto mentioned in an earlier chapter: "Grant me the serenity to accept what cannot be changed, the courage to change what can be changed, and the wisdom to know the difference."

COMPLIMENTING THE STAFF

Because of the depth of feelings that surround nursing-home problems, and because family members are so busy looking for solutions, families may overlook the need to compliment the staff when care is good. Everyone needs recognition for good work, so try to remember to express your appreciation to the staff when you feel they are trying. *You* know what a difficult job it can be to care for a repetitious, confused older person, so let the staff know that you value them. If their work is really exceptional, be sure to let their supervisor or the administrator know, as this can be a real incentive to better performance for all the staff. And paying compliments is much easier than complaining.

VISITING

Visiting in a nursing home can be particularly difficult for the relatives of the mentally impaired older person. Unaware of his whereabouts, your kin may recognize you and be happy with your visit, but he may forget that you were there five minutes later. Or he may be upset when he recognizes you, reproaching you for putting him in a nursing home. He may recognize you but confuse you with someone else in the family. If you remind him of who you are, he may insist, "You're not my daughter. She's dead." Or your relative may have stopped speaking altogether.

These are some of the things that make visiting very difficult. You must work out for yourself how to structure your
visits so that they will be more pleasurable.

Many relatives ask how often they should visit. Some
visit daily, some as seldom as once a month. But most
family members who live within traveling distance visit
from once to three times weekly. How can you decide how
often to visit?

If your relative forgets that you have visited immediately after you leave, once or twice a week is probably
enough, unless *you* need to see him more often. But even
when your relative forgets or is unaware of your visit, it is
important to put in an appearance to let the staff see that
you are concerned about the care your relative is receiving.
How often that type of visit should take place depends
upon your feelings and your assessment of the care.

For most relatives, the problem is not the quantity of
visits but the quality. If you are a regular visitor, if you get
to know the staff and other patients and their families, the
experience can be a pleasurable, sociable one. If you are
able to overcome the pain caused by your relative's condition and enjoy a sense of purpose in visiting, it can also be
enriching. One relative I recall vividly was a devoted
daughter who was unable to accept her mother's mental
condition and felt she should visit every day. She would
visit every other patient on the floor, getting satisfaction
from their appreciation of her, but was unable to spend
more than a few minutes with her own mother.

Others are able to maintain old ways of relating, in
spite of mental deterioration, or are inventive in finding
ways to pass time together. Remember, it's not necessary
to have sensible conversations if this is beyond your relative's ability. You do not have to entertain your kin. You

do not have to provide news about the family, or discuss current events if your relative no longer understands what's going on in the family or the world. You simply have to demonstrate your feeling for your relative— through words, facial expression, or embraces. Sometimes it's enough to sit and hold hands.

Some families find that they can make their visits more pleasant by going for walks or outings, provided that a change of environment is not upsetting to their kin. Looking at pictures or listening to familiar music can also be pleasant. The occupational therapist might suggest simple projects or games that your relative will be able to manage. Reminiscing can be delightful if your kin can still recall past events—and many do, even though they may be totally confused about the present. Family albums can be a source of pleasure, but they can be upsetting if your relative is very confused. Determine what works through trial and error.

Should your relative be brought home for dinners or family events? Only if it still has meaning for you and your relative. Sometimes families make arrangements with the nursing home to take their relatives home for dinner, only to find that they are very restless and anxious to get back to their new home. You may feel hurt or rejected if this happens, but remember that your kin probably can't handle too much mental stimulation or changes in environment. He probably feels safer remaining in his new environment, and you must learn to accept this and not take it personally.

The most important principles influencing how often to visit, and the nature of the visits, should be your feelings, your availability, your relative's response, and the need to demonstrate your concern to the staff.

WHEN YOUR RELATIVE IMPROVES

Sometimes an older person improves after adjusting to life in the nursing home, despite a diagnosis of irreversible brain failure. Nutritious regular meals, a new medication regimen, good nursing care, and the increased stimulation of new people in a new environment all might lead to an improved level of functioning or an improved mood. If your relative lived with you prior to nursing-home placement, you may find yourself bothered by ambivalent feelings. Part of you might rejoice over the improvement, but part of you might feel envious of the nursing-home staff for succeeding where you failed. You may be angry with the staff if they bring out warm and friendly responses from your kin; you may feel that they have displaced you in the affections of your loved one. At the same time you may feel grateful for whatever happiness your kin experiences in his new home. If it's your spouse who is in the institution, you may actually feel jealous if you see him smiling and responsive to the nurses or aides, or holding hands with another resident. Prepare yourself for these possibilities, because they're common.

Remind yourself that the nursing home can become a new social world for the mentally impaired. There are many new relationship opportunities—with residents, nurses, aides, housekeeping staff, therapists, dietary workers, and others—and communication takes many forms. Residents from different cultures (sometimes speaking different languages) can relate to each other at a level of friendship that only they understand. Thus, the nursing-home environment, which may be depressing to you, may prove to be favorable to your kin.

On occasion, residents may improve with care to such

an extent that they insist they don't belong in the nursing home and may plead with visitors to take them home. I remember one resident with very severe memory loss who had been admitted to a nursing home after setting a few accidental fires. She had never been able to accept supervision and had suffered from neglect at home. She responded well to the therapeutic milieu of the nursing home and seemed so intact that she was very convincing during a psychiatric interview, saying "You're the psychiatrist. Just get me out of here." But she couldn't recall anything she did or said even within a few minutes of leaving the interview. She still needed a protective environment.

Sometimes, however, an impaired older person becomes more manageable on an appropriate medication regimen; therefore, apartments and furnishings should not be disposed of too quickly. A return to the community with supervision by a health-care team should certainly be tried. Unfortunately, at the present time most communities are not prepared to offer a continuum of care, tailoring the amount of services to the needs of the old person, which may vary from time to time.

Many old people are locked into the nursing-home system once admitted, or are transferred to other institutions providing lower levels of care, simply because the current system of long-term care does not offer adequate choices for the impaired older person and his family. Many issues now being studied by social and health planners are confused by concerns about the cost of care, which is realistic, but not in relation to the total needs of the chronically impaired. This is a major social policy issue currently being researched and debated, to be solved someday, it is hoped, but not in time to make it easier for you and your kin.

WHEN YOUR RELATIVE GETS WORSE

Sometimes one sees a rapid deterioration after a relative enters a home. Or the relative may remain stable for a long time, and then suddenly show evidence of physical and mental decline. What issues surface at this time?

Most families want to know what is causing the change in condition. Usually the charge nurse is able to give enough information for you to feel that everything that should be done is being done. You should be aware that in most nursing homes it is the charge nurse who assumes major responsibility for the patient's health care. The physician, who is legally responsible for the patient's care, often writes orders based upon information given to him by the nurses.

If you feel that your relative's deterioration may be related to some treatable condition (other than that which is causing the mental deterioration), discuss it with the physician. It is not always easy to get to talk to the physician about your relative's condition, since doctors are usually protected by the nursing staff. But you have a right to talk directly to the doctor, even though you will probably have to arrange an appointment with him through the nurse.

When faced with specific medical problems, you should not be left wondering whether your relative is being treated adequately or neglected. Be aware of his condition and the treatment possibilities. Then the question can legitimately be raised as to how much medical intervention is appropriate. This is a profound issue of values and ethics, and it is a relatively new one, since medical science can now keep chronically impaired people alive indefinitely. It is an issue you wouldn't have had to face twenty years ago, when your relative would have died of natural causes like pneumonia, appendicitis, or ordinary accidents.

Some families are not able to accept the possibility of the death of their loved ones without the reassurance that all means have been used to keep them alive as long as humanly possible. Others are more upset by the quality of life for their impaired kin and are quite clear in their determination not to permit "heroic measures" or highly technical medical treatment to extend their relatives' lives. The question has been posed, "Does intervention prolong life or does it prolong dying?"

Chapter 13 will examine the issues affecting the terminal stage of life, where death is foreseeable. But as an issue in the nursing home, it is important to explore your feelings when requesting or refusing medical intervention for your kin.

Whatever your point of view, you will have to live with the consquences of your decisions. As far as possible, try to sort through your emotions and seek the answers to some questions that may lead you to rational decision-making. What will be the quality of life remaining to my relative if medical treatment keeps him alive? Will he be aware of being alive or not? If he were capable of understanding the dilemma, what would he choose? If I were in his situation, what would I want done for me? An alert, intelligent resident of a geriatric center in which I worked, arguing against medical intervention in the event of terminal illness, put it this way: "When the sphincter fails to sphinct, who wants to be around for the ensuing mess?"

Too often, family members who have not been able to work through their guilt for placing their relative in a home may demand unreasonable levels of treatment for a patient who is clearly ready to die. If the impaired older person no longer wants to eat, for example, might it not be a signal that his life has run its course? Is it ethical to force food into him or to insist on nourishment through tube-feeding? For whose benefit is it? For the uneasy conscience of the family? For the institution? Or for the dying old patient?

As more and more families face these issues and have the opportunity to talk them over with counselors, clergy, and other families, they will find it somewhat easier to raise them with the medical staff.

12

Support Groups

When I developed the first training program for families of the mentally impaired aged, I thought of it as a modest project, one that might help a few people deal with these problems and possibly lead to better treatment of the mentally impaired older person. What I really wanted to do was develop a special facility for the mentally impaired aged to show how they could be cared for more humanely and reasonably by emphasizing special ongoing training for the staff. This was not a feasible project, I learned, for it is very difficult to introduce methods that do not fit into the structure already in operation.

The training program grew from an awareness that the family, which is potentially the most significant part of the system caring for the impaired, also needs training in fulfilling its appropriate role, whether its relative is in the community or in an institution. What I learned from the program, and from subsequent groups, was that the most important aspect of the meetings was the opportunity for the family members to get together, to talk about their feelings, and to draw comfort and strength from one another.

What I thought at first was a modest program turned out to be a very valuable method for people in pain to find some relief. The learning content of the program was helpful, but even more helpful and satisfying were the relationships that developed among people with mutual concerns. When asked if the group was helpful, one member spoke for many. She said, "It sure is. I guess this proves that misery loves company." When the program became a support group that met on a monthly basis, many said that looking forward to the next meeting with their new-found friends helped them get through the month.

Since mental impairment can be expected to last for many years, you, the family, must plan a strategy for coping. Many of the friends and relatives who are supportive at first will drop out, not being able to bear the painful decline or the nonstop sorrow. Finding a suppport group of families going through similar problems can be an enormous help to you.

Family groups are able to listen to stories of how difficult it is to relate to a mentally impaired relative. In fact, they *want* to hear them. They can find humor in them, or they can cry together, but they can handle it. Their strength as a group carries over to the individual. It's one of the best methods I know of for dealing with this chronic condition.

In recent years, groups have been formed all over the country through the Alzheimer's Disease and Related Disorders Association, as mentioned in chapter 4 (see Appendix 3 for the address of the national headquarters and its toll-free phone number). This organization has chapters in many cities, which can tell you about local groups of relatives of mentally impaired older persons.

You can also look for support groups through your local mental health association, YMCA or YWCA, office for the aging, or geriatric centers; there are also religiously affiliated and nonsectarian family service agencies that sponsor groups. A recent directory of family support groups has been compiled by the National Support Center for Families of the Aging, P.O. Box 245, Swarthmore, Pennsylvania 19081.

If there are no groups available in your area, you should look into starting one on your own. It is not hard to do if you have the time and energy to make a few phone calls. The book *The 36-Hour Day*, by Nancy Mace and Peter Rabins, contains an excellent section on how to start a group, with guidelines on how to conduct them. (See the list of recommended reading at the end of this book.)

One potential place for finding family groups or starting them is a nursing home. Although at present I know of no groups that include family members of patients in the institution as well as those whose kin are in the community, this is a logical and helpful combination. If you propose this possibility to administrators of local nursing homes as a means of helping families adjust to their role in the institution, while preparing families for these possibilities in the community, you may be successful in getting their cooperation.

Through a support group, you can also learn new ways of coping, sharing information about resources, and developing ways of negotiating with your local network of services. Where services don't exist, you might make your local needs known to advocacy groups, such as the Gray Panthers, the American Association of Retired Persons, or local senior citizen centers. As you meet more people who are going through the same problems you are facing, you will get new ideas about what services are needed and how to go about getting them.

FAMILY COUNCILS

Most good nursing homes have established family councils, but some administrators are still afraid to encourage their development. As families become more knowledgeable about these issues, they should try to find someone on staff who might help them to begin a council. All that is needed are a few relatives who can volunteer to contact other families, and the cooperation of the nursing-home administrator in providing a room for the meetings. Since most visits to the nursing home take place on Saturday or Sunday, it is generally best to plan meetings for one of those days. The hours of one to three P.M. are most popular. Of course, conditions vary from one area to another, and groups have to work out for themselves the most convenient time for meetings.

A family council can provide a legitimate, significant role within the nursing home for the relatives, making it easier for them to learn about the institution and to identify which problems are unique to their kin and which are common to many. It is more efficient for staff to listen to one relative as a representative of a group, rather than to take time to listen to many relatives with the same problems, and it is easier for the relatives to present problems as a group, since their complaints are less likely to be interpreted by the staff as personal criticism.

Family councils have been described by the eminent sociologist Eugene Litwak of Columbia University as linkage mechanisms that function to balance and coordinate the special needs of the families and the staffs in large organizations. This balance must be found in order to achieve their shared goal of good care for the individual by the institution. Just as parent-teacher organizations can lead to improvement in the quality of education in the schools, a family council can encourage better-quality care in an institution.

If it proves to be too difficult to start a family council within the institution, look for an outside organization that addresses itself to the families of patients in nursing homes. For example, in New York there is Friends and Relatives of the Institutionalized Aged (FRIA), which brings together relatives from many different nursing homes. They have become advocates for better care for patients, and they bring their problems to the attention of individual nursing-home administrators and to governmental regulatory agencies when they feel it is necessary.

There are advantages and disadvantages to this type of organization. Because they function outside the institution, their representatives are often viewed as adversaries by administrators. This can lead to resistance to suggestions for improving conditions. However, it can also lead to results if the group has sufficient clout and the administrators have reason to fear inquiries by regulatory agencies. Nonetheless, it is more difficult for a family council to function without the base of a host institution, since the problems discussed by the members will vary considerably because of differences between individual nursing homes. It is also much more difficult for members to learn the facts, since they don't have easy access to the lines of communication in all of the nursing homes represented. Some families, however, prefer to use the anonymity of an outside organization to air their complaints, fearing to antagonize the staff in their own nursing home by direct discussion.

DAY-CARE CENTERS

Urgently needed by families in the community are day-care centers prepared to serve the mentally impaired older person. There are only a few such facilities in the entire country.

If you and other family members feel that day care might meet some of your needs, you might try to organize your own, just as working mothers of preschool children have been successful in starting such programs. What you need first is the commitment of a few people with varied experience to plan and develop a program. You will need a place to provide care for ten to twenty people, in order to make it financially feasible. You may find a church, synagogue, school, library, or other public facility that will give you some space. Look for help from local women's or men's fraternal or civic groups, such as the Odd Fellows, Kiwanis, or Masons, to name a few. They represent a vast amount of experience that may be tapped for a social cause, both in planning and in implementing your program.

You will then need the help of a lawyer (donated, if possible) to incorporate you as a nonprofit organization so that you will be exempt from taxes, eligible for grants, and protected from lawsuits. You must become aware of local and state regulations and get sound advice about insurance and liability.

You should find someone with business experience who can help to develop a budget. The staff should include one or two supervisors (with a background in nursing, social work, teaching, or recreation, and with specialized knowledge in the care of the mentally impaired aged) and a number of aides, depending upon how many impaired persons are registered for the program. It will be very important to recruit volunteers to work with the staff, to keep costs manageable, and to meet the diverse needs of the group. Family members of the impaired may find it more gratifying to volunteer to work for a day or a half-day with a group than to spend all their time with a relative.

Programs should be worked out according to the capacities of the group, but generally they should include such physical activities as modified exercises, music sessions, and simple crafts. A care plan for each impaired older person should be approved by his own physician. The possibilities are limitless, depending on the resources available and on the experience, imagination, and creativity of the staff, family, and volunteers.

At the present time this type of program must be privately funded, supported by a grant, or voluntarily run, since it does not fall under any existing category of service that is eligible for coverage. However, since the program would be developed to meet a health need, efforts should be made to explore the possibility of government funding. Mental impairment *is* an illness.

Some health insurance plans pay for home health care under certain conditions, and there is widespread concern about the high cost of care in institutions. Therefore, since the cost of day care would be much lower than that of institutionalization, and since day care can be an alternative to institutional care—at least temporarily—the time may be ripe for families of the mentally impaired aged to press for such programs to be covered by government funds or health insurance.

Although such urgently needed programs do not exist as yet, and although funding is not available under current regulations, a grass roots movement to lobby for specialized day care may indeed have some political impact. It is said that one major reason that Medicare came about was that President Eisenhower learned about the high cost of health care when his mother-in-law became ill, and pressed the congressional committee formulating the legislation to rush it through. In the same way, the need for specialized day care for the mentally impaired aged may be recognized as more and more legislators experience the problem in their own families.

SITTERS' COOPERATIVES

For a more immediate solution, sometimes an informal sharing arrangement of daytime care for a few hours with other families can offer considerable relief. Five or six impaired persons can be cared for in the home of one family member for several hours, or a whole day, in exchange for an equal amount of time from other members of the group. In this way, a "sitters' cooperative" can be started, with no financial outlay. Members can share ideas with one another for projects that can be effective in providing the most appropriate care in the home.

These may seem like unrealistic suggestions, given your day-to-day burdens, but if the time expended in planning should result in a day-care program six months from now, or a sitters' cooperative in the near future, wouldn't it be worth the effort?

All of these programs, either paid for or based on an exchange of services, can come from the contacts of a support group, or can lead to the formation of a support group. Whichever comes first, you will find that the members of your support group can be the most important source of help in getting you through this dark time.

A Timely Death

Most people don't like to think about death, but families of the mentally impaired aged find themselves thinking about it quite often, sometimes even wishing for it. And they find themselves feeling terribly guilty and remorseful for the morbid thoughts.

The psychology of death and dying is a very recent field of study. Professionals working with the dying and their families are just beginning to recognize that they must become aware of their *own* feelings before they can help others with their grief. In the same way I think it can be helpful for families to recognize the complexity of *their* feelings in trying to cope with the mental death of someone they care about while waiting for physical death to catch up.

ACCEPTANCE

Most healthy people don't want to die. Even if we overcome our fears to the extent that we can accept its inevitability, we still don't want it to happen to us. Even those who are sustained by a religious belief in the hereafter or in the immortality of the soul don't want to die. Why? Dying is the end of all we care about, the loss of everyone we love, the loss of ourselves.

This is such a fundamentally terrifying experience that it is no wonder it's shrouded in mystery. As soon as someone dies, he is no longer a person. He is a body, a corpse, and he's removed as quickly as possible. There are rituals for handling a corpse and burying it. The funeral director refers to "the remains" of the deceased. It is dreadful to think of ourselves as "remains," so we tend to avoid thinking about our own death, and prefer not thinking about death in general.

One way of handling our anxieties is to treat them with humor. There are endless jokes about death, almost as many as there are about sex. A movie impresario who was still working and making a fortune in his mid-eighties was asked, "Why do you work so hard? You know you can't take it with you." He answered, "I'm not going!" And then there's the story of the old man on his deathbed who whispers to his son keeping vigil, "I can smell Mama's apple strudel baking in the kitchen. I would like one last taste before I die. Ask her for a little piece." The son comes back empty-handed, saying, "Mama says it's for after the funeral."

The mentally alert aged use lots of humor in coping with whatever fears they may have about dying. I remember one ninety-two-year-old resident of a geriatric center who, when his subscription to a weekly news magazine was running out, asked me, "Should I renew for one year, or should I gamble and take the bargain rate for three years?" And I remember one applicant to the center who said, "I'm at that stage of life where I wear my prettiest nightgown every night when I go to bed, in case someone has to find me in the morning."

The quips and lighthearted banter often used by the elderly when talking about their age and future indicate their acceptance of their mortality. They are a very good sign.

But the ability to accept death calls paradoxically for the ability to accept our life as it is and as it has been. One of the final tasks that faces us in the last stage of life is the acceptance of our life as it has been. If we are beset with a sense of unfulfillment, feelings of remorse for things undone or unspoken, then we have not successfully worked through this necessary task in achieving a satisfactory old age. One way that older people are able to accomplish this task is through the process of life review, as identified by Dr. Robert Butler, one of our country's foremost authorities on aging. Through reminiscing one is able to reaffirm the positive aspects of his past life and understand the reasons for the failures and disappointments. Through the life-review process one can validate his existence by accepting the past, integrating both good and bad. If there is a sense of unhappiness, the older person can be encouraged to do whatever still can be done to change things so that he works toward acceptance and lives to the fullest until he dies.

The inability of a mentally impaired older person to joke about death or to engage in this process of life review places an additional burden on the relative who witnesses the slow death without the sense of completion that can come with acceptance.

The care-giving relatives who have assumed the role of protectors may find themselves trying to work through this mental process of acceptance in lieu of their kin, who can no longer find meaning in life. This can be extremely stressful, for how can a surrogate find a life acceptable that ends with such indignities?

This may give us a clue to one source of the turmoil that is felt by the relatives who cannot help but wish that death would end their burden. Apparently there are times we can wish for death when life is no longer acceptable, but although we wish for death, it is also not truly acceptable because the life that is ending is not acceptable. One technique for resolving this painful conflict is to accept the life of the impaired older person as it was until the beginning of the deteriorating illness. The period of severe mental impairment marks a state of limbo. It is no longer representative of the life of the older person; it is part of the process of dying. When viewed in this context, the condition of mental impairment forces a direct confrontation with death; when it finally arrives, death may be less painful, since it can be viewed as the end of a dying process.

Is death ever really accepted? Of course it is. We all know of people who have died a "good death," serenely, at peace with themselves. What constitutes a good death?

Many old people have learned to accept death by virtue of years of practice at accepting losses. Advanced old age brings the loss of many friends and relatives, and many adjustments must be made. Changes in oneself are also viewed as losses, as one's social world shrinks in relation to physical limitations, reduced capacities, weariness. Indeed, at times death is not only acceptable to the very old, frail person; it can be desirable. The comment "It's time to go; I'm ready" does not necessarily signify sadness. It can be a statement of acceptance. But it can also be a sign of resignation, a call for help in working through unresolved emotions until acceptance can be achieved.

We talk of death in many dimensions—a fast death, a difficult death, an easy death, a timely death, an untimely death. When someone of very advanced years dies, in some ways it is a timely death, to be expected as a natural event; yet for those who deeply love the deceased, death is never timely. The moment of death is always experienced as a shock.

I sat next to an aged woman on a park bench not long ago. She told me that recently she had lost her husband, and she talked at length about what a shock it was and how she would never be able to recover from it. Thinking that some comfort might be drawn from the fact that they had lived many years together, I asked gently, "How old was he?" "He was ninety-four," she said. "But he was never sick. Not one day in the hospital. Just suddenly dropped dead. I'll never get over it." For the widow, his death was not timely.

Our ability to accept death as timely may be based partly on having time—a period of illness—to prepare for it, to anticipate the grief that will be felt, and to start to mourn. The duration of terminal illness in old age and the awareness by the patient of his condition will influence how the family prepares for the inevitable loss. If the illness has caused the patient pain and fear, the family can more easily accept the death as a blessing. If it has gone on for a long time, death can be viewed as a release, for which the family has already partially mourned. If it goes on for more than a few months, the death can be thought of as overdue, and at least privately wished for by the emotionally drained and grieving family.

Caring for a mentally impaired older person has been compared to a funeral without an end, but it is much more painful than a funeral. A funeral provides the opportunity to release our emotions in the company of family and friends, and it lasts only a few hours. But the period of caring for the mentally impaired lasts much longer, and there's limited support from family and friends. It is much, much worse than a funeral. It is bereavement with no end in sight.

THE DYNAMICS OF GRIEF

Our understanding of grief as a process has been clarified through the work of Dr. Eric Lindemann, who in 1944 studied the effect of a catastrophe on the survivors of the victims. Although the victims were not elderly, his observations about the patterns of reaction of the survivors are applicable to many families of the aged. The first pattern he identified was physical distress, such as sighing, shortness of breath, digestive disturbances, and exhaustion. The second was a preoccupation with the image of the deceased. The third pattern he found was guilt, with a sense of personal responsibility for the death of the loved one, expressed as regrets for things the survivors should have done. The fourth pattern was feelings of anger, and the fifth and last was confusion over the loss of the survivors' normal pattern of conduct.

In coping with these symptoms and feelings, Lindemann found that five basic tasks must be accomplished to overcome grief. This process has been called "grief work."

1. "Dealing with the pain of facing the loss." One must be allowed to cry and to express inner desperation.

2. "All of the emotions, such as fear, anger, guilt, must be experienced." They must be talked out.

3. "Eventually by admitting the separation through death, the grieving person must be free from bondage to the deceased." Guilt must be overcome, and preoccupation with the image of the deceased must yield to other concerns.

4. "A grieving person must ultimately readjust to the social environment." This calls for giving up old roles and behaviors and assuming new ones.

5. "New relationships must be formulated." If the loss is of a very significant member of the social support system, replacements must be found.

When the grief you experience is anticipatory, prior to the death of your loved one, you go through these stages a little at a time, but your feelings are just as intense. The relative of a severely mentally impaired older person grieves over the mental death of his loved one while the physical being lingers on. The essence of the person no longer exists, but the body remains. Sometimes it is as though a different person were occupying the structure of the person who no longer exists, and while the former person is mourned, the new and different person, demanding care and attention, does not allow the mourning to be resolved.

This part of the process can be called partial grief.

Since the bereaved relative still has the presence of the mentally impaired older person to contend with, he can cry and talk about his emotions, but he cannot yet free himself from bondage. He may be partially readjusting to his environment, but the adjustments are not necessarily bringing satisfying new roles. Grief must be worked through in stages, gradually putting distance between the past and the anguish of the present. Effective grief work requires the suspension of regular roles. Time away from normal tasks is needed to cry out the pain and to do the talking necessary to find order in past recollections and take stock of the present and future.

You can see how the relative of a mentally impaired older person can have a much more difficult time in bereavement than the survivor of someone who has died. At least the survivor can go through a normal period of preparatory grief and mourning, finally achieving some detachment and easing of pain.

THE IMPACT OF BEREAVEMENT

The bereavement of someone who loses a spouse is different from the bereavement of someone who loses a parent. When a spouse dies, the survivor enters a new status, as widow or widower, and the new status carries expectations for behavior, including the opportunity to grieve and then to establish the new identities. How this is handled depends upon the quality and length of the marriage, the survivor's ability to cope, and the support available to the one who is grieving. But this grief is very difficult to face before the death actually occurs. The emptiness and loneliness, and the confusion over how to take on new roles, sometimes cannot be confronted in advance.

When an adult prepares for the death of a parent, it is also experienced as a crisis, even though it may be a normal transition, to be expected. As in the case of a spouse, the intensity of loss will depend upon the quality of the parent-child relationship. But whether the relationship was predominantly positive or largely negative, the death of a parent will be profoundly felt by the adult child. There is no new status for the adult who loses a parent—whoever heard of an aging orphan?—yet one may feel like an orphan, alone and abandoned.

The most frequent emotional response common to both is a mixture of guilt and anger. For a spouse, there is guilt for being the survivor when your partner is dying. (You might spare yourself the guilt if you remind yourself that your turn will come.) Then, there is anger at being left alone. For the adult child, there is guilt for not preventing the death of a parent, perhaps even for wishing for the death, and anger for being put through such pain. Then comes more guilt for being selfish enough to be angry. If they are not recognized, these emotions can lead to unreasonable reactions regarding the care of your kin. If you have allowed yourself to wish for death, you may fear unconsciously that this wish caused the death of your loved one. In your panic not to cause the death, you may go to extremes in seeking treatment that will prevent death.

You must remind yourself constantly that no one, including you yourself, is the cause of your relative's condition. When death occurs, it will be caused by a combination of conditions that are related to the mental impairment.

In a previous chapter, the issue of medical intervention in the event of terminal illness of residents in nursing homes was discussed. The issue applies as well to those whose kin are in the community. It was not too long ago that pneumonia was called "the old man's friend." Modern medicine now commonly postpones death for the chronically impaired old person by curing the intervening illnesses. If death is imminent, however, the family might discuss with the physician whether further treatment is appropriate or whether it would be better to let nature take its course. If the family is able to face this dilemma with a physician who knows the history of the patient's chronic condition, a decision can be reached that is ethical, humane, and just for all concerned.

You may have come to accept the idea of the actual death of your kin as preferable to the continuation of this living death, but at a deeper level you may not be ready for the total bereavement that awaits you. You may feel that you should be warding off death, protecting your relative, who can no longer care for himself.

Consider, then, what your loved one would want if he were competent to understand his situation. Most alert older people state emphatically that they are not afraid to die and that they would rather die than suffer senility. Old age is no blessing if it is spent in the befuddled or disturbed netherworld of senility. What you really want is to abolish senility, to cure brain failure. But for that there is no cure, at least not yet.

Remind yourself that you are not omnipotent. By accepting death you can be better prepared to allow death when the time comes without blaming yourself or others. If you have to place blame somewhere, blame fate. Again, and still again, seek the serenity to accept what you cannot change, the courage to change what can be changed, and the wisdom to know the difference.

APPENDIX 1

Safety, Health, and Nutritional Needs for Mentally Impaired Older Persons Living Alone

1. Make sure that your relative is safe, by personal observation and/or by checking with neighbors, the postman, or grocery store clerk that:
   a) he is dressing appropriately
   b) he is capable of locking and unlocking the door
   c) he is not wandering off
   d) he is walking steadily
   e) he is using stove and other appliances safely
   f) he is capable of handling cigarettes
2. Check on your relative's health by:
   a) consulting regularly with an interested physician
   b) verifying whether medications ordered are taken properly by counting pills

    c) personally observing that hygiene is adequate and sanitary conditions are maintained

    d) observing signs of depression, consulting with doctor as to whether treatable

3. Check on nutrition by:

    a) periodically verifying food purchases and methods of preparation

    b) inspecting refrigerator, garbage can, cupboards, closets

    c) checking weight regularly and observing energy level

    d) controlling alcohol supply if relative drinks

4. If you suspect that your relative has become incapable of adequate self-care in the above areas, you must:

    a) arrange for home help

or b) provide for the care yourself

or c) have someone else in the family do so

or d) move your relative to the home of someone in the family, or move your relative to a supervised setting

APPENDIX 2

Principles for Managing a Mentally Impaired Older Person in Your Home

1. Consult with the Visiting Nurse Service or Home Health Agency about safety, health, and nutritional standards. Watch for potential hazards and avoid them as the capacity of the older person changes. Protect your relative and others with effective locks on doors and safety devices on the stove, and by putting medications out of reach, protecting valuables, supervising bathing, etc.

2. Accept the new mental function of your relative as realistically assessed by a physician, and anticipate resulting behavior. Accept your relative as a different person, toward whom you must assume different roles, although

the relationship remains the same. Don't cause unnecessary stress by placing excessive demands. Ignore upsetting behavior, if possible. Recognize repetitious questions and clinging behavior as signs of insecurity. Use logic when trying to understand the meaning of sentences when words are missing or misused. Be imaginative. Guess what your relative might want to tell you. Get him to show what he wants, without verbal language. Search for the feelings he is trying to express—fear, anger, love—and let him know you understand, which can minimize frustration. Try to be patient, calm, and reassuring. Try to express caring with words and embraces. Be vigilant and protective.

3. Accept the new reality of your kin. Don't argue and use facts and logic to try to prove he is wrong. Be prepared to shift your stance in a discussion to avoid unnecessary outbursts. Try to orient your relative to reality, but be flexible when his reality has changed. Invent an acceptable story, if necessary, to reassure him and ensure appropriate care, focusing on the positive purpose of the fiction. Use compromise as a technique to reduce tension. Forgive yourself when you lose patience.

4. Provide a structured, calm routine as much as possible. Get ideas from as many sources as possible for activities that might occupy your relative. Play music if he enjoys it and if it doesn't cause additional confusion.

5. Assume only as much control as needed. Allow as much personal choice and decision as possible. Don't treat your impaired relative like a baby, but provide firm discipline when necessary. Try to understand the feelings of

your relative as expressed by his behavior, and tell him what you think he is feeling.

6. Get as much help as possible. Don't feel guilty about spending your relative's money for paid help if he has the financial means. Don't begrudge spending your own money for help if you have it. Get help through Medicaid if eligible. Don't be bashful about asking everyone in the family to pitch in with time and money. Don't feel they should know what you need without having to ask; just ask matter-of-factly without reproaches, if possible. Don't be a martyr or a scapegoat. You have enough troubles as it is. Try to arrange to get away regularly.

7. Be prepared for other arrangements such as an alternative relative or institution, if care becomes more than you can handle physically or emotionally.

APPENDIX 3

Directory of Resources

S ervices for the elderly are provided by a variety of public and private agencies, which are subject to political influence and change so rapidly that it is not possible to provide you with an accurate listing of resources that will still be current by the date of publication. I have therefore prepared a guide that should help you begin to locate the services you need in your own community. Don't become discouraged by the many phone calls you may have to make before you find the appropriate agency for your needs.

A first step that may be your best shortcut is a call to

your local chapter of the Alzheimer's Disease and Related Disorders Association. You can find this by calling the toll-free national number 800-621-0379. The address of the national headquarters is 360 North Michigan Avenue, Chicago, Illinois 60601. The members of this organization are committed to sharing information about physicians, social workers, homemakers and attendants, and the range of services needed by families of the mentally impaired aged. Their information, however, is based upon personal experiences, and is therefore not always reliable in other cases.

Most people seeking help about social and health problems are directed to agencies that offer information and referrals to appropriate services. The following list can give you some ideas as to how to locate such an information and referral office in your own area. Most of these offices provide information on a wide range of problems, not necessarily related to the aging. The telephones are often answered by trained volunteers, not professionals. They can usually direct you to appropriate services for the elderly.

SELECTED INFORMATION AND REFERRAL SERVICES

Alabama

BIRMINGHAM
Volunteer and Information Center of Greater Birmingham, Inc.
3600 Eighth Avenue S.
Birmingham 35222

MONTGOMERY
Montgomery Area United Way
P.O. Box 6135
Montgomery 36106

Arizona

FLAGSTAFF
Coconino County Information and Referral
113 West Clay
Flagstaff 86001

PHOENIX
Community Information and Referral Services, Inc.
1515 East Osborn Road
Phoenix 85104

TUCSON
Information and Referral Services, Inc.
2302 East Speedway, 210
Tucson 85719

Arkansas

LITTLE ROCK
Crisis Center of Arkansas/Helpline
5904 West Markham
Little Rock 72205

United Way of Pulaski County
P.O. Box 3257
Little Rock 72203

California

FRESNO
Fresno Community Council
325 Crocker Bank Building
Fresno 93721

LOS ANGELES
CRIB (Community Resource Information Bank)
3000 West Sixth Street
Los Angeles 90020

Information and Referral Federation of Los Angeles County, Inc.
3035 North Tyler Avenue
El Monte 91731

SACRAMENTO
Emergency Assistance and Referral Agency
2824 S Street
Sacramento 95816

Senior Information and Referral Service
St. Paul's Center
1012 Fifteenth Street
Sacramento 95814

SAN DIEGO
Guideline
P.O. Box 17720
San Diego 92117

SAN FRANCISCO
United Way, Bay Area
410 Bush Street
San Francisco 94108

Colorado

BOULDER
Volunteer and Informa-
tion Center of Boulder
County
1823 Folsom, Room 101
Boulder 80302

LONGMONT
Longmont Information
and Referral
525 Fourth Avenue,
Room 225
Longmont 80501

DENVER
Mile High United Way:
Information and Refer-
ral Service
1245 East Colfax,
Room 311
Denver 80218

PUEBLO
United Way of Pueblo
County, Inc.
229 Colorado Avenue
Pueblo 81001

Connecticut

DARIEN
Darien United Way and
Community Council, Inc.
P.O. Box 926
24 Old Kings Highway, S.
Darien 06820

EASTERN REGION
Info Line of Middlesex
County
27 Washington Street
Middletown 06457

GREENWICH
Community Answers
101 West Putnam Avenue
Greenwich 06830

NORTHEASTERN REGION
Info Line Northeast
United Social and Men-
tal Health Services
51 Westcott Road
Danielson 06239

NORTHWESTERN REGION
Info Line
130 Freight Street
Waterbury 06702

NORWALK
Greater Norwalk Com-
munity Council
P.O. Box 2033
Norwalk 06852

NEW HAVEN
South Central Area Info
  Line
1 State Street
New Haven 06511

SOUTHEASTERN REGION
Info Line of Southeastern
  Connecticut
P.O. Box 375
Gales Ferry 06335

WESTPORT
Information and Referral
  Service
Town Hall
Westport 06880

Delaware

NEW CASTLE
Delaware Information
  and Referral Service
"T" Building
Delaware State Hospital
New Castle 19720

District of Columbia
Friendship House Associ-
  ation
619 D Street, S. E.
Washington 20003

Florida

FORT LAUDERDALE
Health and Social Service
  Information and Refer-
  ral Community Service
Council of Broward
  County, Inc.
1300 South Andrews
  Avenue
Fort Lauderdale 33335

GAINESVILLE
Alachua County Crisis
  Center
606 Southwest Third
  Avenue
Gainesville 36201

JACKSONVILLE
Central Crisis Center of
  Jackonsville, Inc.
2218 Park Street
Jacksonville 32204

MIAMI
Department of Human
  Resources
Elderly Services Division
140 W. Flagler Street,
  Suite 1605
Miami 33103

ORLANDO

Information and Referral
  Center
Department of Human
  Services Planning Council
3191 Maguire Boulevard,
  Suite 209
Orlando 32803

Georgia

ATLANTA

United Way of Metropoli-
  tan Atlanta
100 Edgewood Avenue
  Northeast
Atlanta 30303

AUGUSTA

United Way of Richmond-
  Columbia-Lincoln
  Counties and North
  Augusta, Inc.
630 Ellis Street
Augusta 30902

SAVANNAH

United Way Savannah
  Area
P.O. Box 9119
Savannah 31412

Hawaii

HONOLULU

Volunteer Information
  and Referral Service
200 North Vineyard
  Boulevard, Suite 603
Honolulu 96817

Idaho

BOISE

Information and Referral
  Service
1365 North Orchard,
  Suite 107
Boise 83706

IDAHO FALLS

Idaho Falls Regional In-
  formation and Referral
  Services
P.O. Box 2246
Idaho Falls 83401

POCATELLO

Southeastern Idaho Com-
  munity Action Agency
  Information and Refer-
  ral Service
1356 North Main
Pocatello 83201

Illinois

CHICAGO
Community Referral
  Service
64 East Jackson
  Boulevard
Chicago 60604

PEORIA
Information and Referral
  Service
B Level, Public Library
  Building
107 Northeast Monroe
Peoria 61602

ROCKFORD
CONTACT Rockford
P.O. Box 1976
Rockford 61110

United Way Services, Inc.
304 North Main Street
P.O. Box 179
Rockford 61105

SPRINGFIELD
Information and Referral
  Service
730 East Vine Street
  P.O. Box 316
Springfield 62705

Indiana

INDIANAPOLIS
Help-Line Information
  and Referral
Community Service
  Council
1828 North Meridian
  Street
Indianapolis 46202

KOKOMO
Volunteer in Community
  Service
320 West Taylor
Kokomo 46901

SOUTH BEND
Voluntary Action Center,
  Inc.
1509 Miami Street
South Bend 46613

TERRE HAUTE
Vigo County Lifeline, Inc.
200 South Sixth Street
Terre Haute 47807

FORT WAYNE AREA
Northeast Area III
  Council on Aging
227 East Washington
  Boulevard
Fort Wayne 46802

Adams County Council
on Aging
804 Mercer
Decatur 46733

Allen County Council
on Aging
233 West Main Street
Fort Wayne 46802

DeKalb County Council
on Aging
Sixth and Jackson
Auburn 46706

Huntington County
Council on Aging
337 Market Street
Huntington 46750

LaGrange County Coun-
cil on Aging
208 North Sycamore
LaGrange 46761

Noble County Council on
Aging
206 South Main Street
P.O. Box 783
Kendallville 46755

Steuben County Council
on Aging
909 West Maumee
Angola 46703

Wells County Council on
Aging
P.O. Box 227
Bluffton 46714

Whitley County Council
on Aging
603 West Van Buren
Columbia City 46725

Iowa

AMES

Open Line, Inc.
P.O. Box 1138
Welch Avenue Station
Ames 50010

CEDAR RAPIDS

Information and Referral
of East Central Iowa
400 Third Avenue South-
east
Cedar Rapids 52401

DES MOINES

United Way of Greater
Des Moines
700 Sixth Avenue
Des Moines 50309

SIOUX CITY

AID (Assistance, Infor-
mation, Direction) Center
722 Nebraska Street
Sioux City 51101

Kansas

TOPEKA
Community Information
  Services
Topeka Public Library
1515 West Tenth Street
Topeka 66604

WICHITA
United Way Information
  and Referral
420 Insurance Building
212 North Market
Wichita 67202

Kentucky

LEXINGTON
Ask Us
268 West Short Street
Lexington 40507

LOUISVILLE
Crisis and Information
  Center
600 South Preston Street
Louisville 40203

NEWPORT
Aging Information and
  Referral Center
59 Carothers Road
Newport 41071

Louisiana

BATON ROUGE
Library Information
  Service
7711 Goodwood
  Boulevard
Baton Rouge 70806

LAFAYETTE
Southwest Louisiana
  Education and Referral
  Center, Inc.
524 Brook Street
P.O. Box 3844
Lafayette 70506

LAKE CHARLES
Helpline
420 Pujo Street
Lake Charles 70601

NEW ORLEANS
Volunteer and Informa-
  tion Agency
Information and Referral
  Service
211 Camp Street,
  Suite 610
New Orleans 70130

Maine

AUGUSTA

Information and Referral
Department of Human
Services
221 State Street
Augusta 04333

Maryland

BALTIMORE

Health and Welfare
Council of Central
Maryland, Inc.
22 Light Street
Baltimore 21202

HAGERSTOWN

Community Service
Council of Washington
County, Inc.
14 Public Square
Hagerstown 21740

Massachusetts

BOSTON

Citizen Information
Service
Department of the State
Secretary
One Ashburton Place,
Room 1611
Boston 02108

United Way of Massa-
chusetts Bay
Information and Referral
Service
87 Kilby Street
Boston 02109

Michigan

DETROIT

TIP Service (The
Information Place)
Detroit Public Library
5201 Woodward
Detroit 48202

Community Information
Services
United Community Ser-
vices of Metropolitan
Detroit
51 West Warren
Detroit 48201

FLINT

Voluntary Action Center
Information and Referral
Service of Genesee and
Lapeer Counties
202 East Boulevard Drive,
Room 330
Flint 48503

GRAND RAPIDS
Information and Referral
  Center of VIA
66 North Division
Grand Rapids 49503

LANSING
Capital Area United Way
300 North Washington
Lansing 48933

Minnesota

DULUTH
Information and Referral
211 West Second Street
Duluth 55802

MINNEAPOLIS
First Call for Help
404 South Eighth Street
Minneapolis 55404

ST. PAUL
Community Planning
  Organization
333 Sibley Street
St. Paul 55101

Mississippi

JACKSON
Allied Services
Aging Division
City of Jackson

326 South Street
Jackson 39201

TUPELO
Lee United Neighbors'
  Information Place
P.O. Box 334
Tupelo 38801

Missouri

KANSAS CITY
The Voluntary Action
  and Information Center
605 West 47th Street,
  Suite 300
Kansas City 64112

ST. LOUIS
United Way Information
  and Referral Service
915 Olive Street
St. Louis 63101

Montana

BILLINGS
District 7
Human Resources
2518 First Avenue North
Billings 59101

HELENA
Montana State Informa-
  tion and Referral Service

(406) 449-5650 or
  (800) 852-3388 (toll free)

Nebraska

LINCOLN
Lincoln Information Ser-
  vice for the Elderly (LIFE)
901 P Street, Room 224
Lincoln 68508

OMAHA
Eastern Nebraska Office
  on Aging
885 South 72nd Street
Omaha 68114

United Way of the
  Midlands
Information and Referral
1805 Harney Street
Omaha 68102

Nevada

LAS VEGAS
Voluntary Action Center
  of Greater Las Vegas
212 East Mequite
Las Vegas 89101

RENO
Voluntary Action Center
790 Sutro Street
Reno 89512

New Hampshire

CONCORD
Concord/Central New
  Hampshire Information
  Outlet
13 South State Street
Concord 03301

KEENE
Monadnock Health and
  Welfare Council
9 Center Street
Keene 03431

New Jersey

ATLANTIC COUNTY
Atlantic County Informa-
  tion and Referral Service
1601 Atlantic Avenue,
  Fifth Floor
Atlantic City 08401

BERGEN COUNTY
Health and Welfare
  Council of Bergen
  County: Information
  and Referral Service
389 Main Street
Hackensack 07601

CAMDEN COUNTY
Contact 609
1050 North Kings

Highway
Cherry Hill 08304

Union Organization for
  Social Services
Community Information
  and Referral Office
211 South Sixth Street
Camden 08103

CENTRAL NEW JERSEY
United Way of Central
  Jersey, Inc.
32 Ford Avenue
P.O. Box 210
Milltown 08850

GLOUCESTER COUNTY
Information and Referral
  of Human Services
  Coalition
P.O. Box 430
Woodbury 08096

HUDSON COUNTY
First Call for Help
857 Bergen Avenue
Jersey City 07306

MERCER COUNTY
Greater Mercer Compre-
  hensive Planning Council
3131 Princeton Pike,
  Building 4
P.O. Box 2103
Trenton 08607

MONMOUTH COUNTY
Community Services
  Council for Monmouth
  County
601 Bangs Avenue,
  Room 503
Asbury Park 07712

MONTCLAIR
North Essex Help-Line
60 South Fullerton
  Avenue
Montclair 07042

MORRIS COUNTY
United Way of Morris
  County
250 James Street
Morristown 07960

NEWARK
United Labor Agency of
  Essex-West Hudson, Inc.
605 Broad Street
Newark 07102

OCEAN COUNTY
First Call for Help
Bishop Memorial Library
Washington Street
Toms River 08753

PRINCETON
First Call for Help
Princeton Area Council of
  Community Services

25 Valley Road
P.O. Box 201
Princeton 08540

SOMERSET
Information Center
Somerset County Library
North Bridge Street and
    Vogt Drive
Bridgewater 08807

New Mexico

ALBUQUERQUE
United Way of Greater
    Albuquerque
P.O. Box 1767
Albuquerque 87103

New York

NEW YORK CITY
Department for Aging
2 Lafayette Street
New York 10007

ALBANY COUNTY
Infoline of Albany
    County
Albany County Court-
    house, Room 315
Albany 12207

BUFFALO AND ERIE
COUNTY
United Way of Buffalo
    and Erie County
742 Delaware Avenue
Buffalo 14209

CHAUTAUQUA COUNTY
Project DIAL
101 West Fifth Street
Jamestown 14701

DUTCHESS COUNTY
Information Line of
    United Way
75 Market Street
Poughkeepsie 12601

ITHACA
Tompkins County Infor-
    mation and Referral
313 Aurora Street
Ithaca 14850

MONTGOMERY COUNTY
Montgomery County
    Department of Social
    Services
County Office Building
Fonda 12068

NASSAU COUNTY
Nassau County Depart-
    ment of Health: In-
    formation and Refer-
    ral Service

240 Old Country Road
Mineola 11501

Nassau County Department of Senior Citizen
Affairs
222 Willis Avenue
Mineola 11501

NIAGARA COUNTY
Action Information
1603 Main Street
Niagara Falls 14305

ONONDAGA COUNTY
Community Service of
the Volunteer Center,
Inc.
Gridley Building,
Fourth Floor
103 Water Street
Syracuse 13202

ORANGE COUNTY
Mental Health Association in Orange County,
Inc.
P.O. Box 238
Goshen 10924

ROCKLAND COUNTY
Rockland County Department of Social Services
Sanatorium Road,
Building L
Pomona 10970

ROME AND WESTERN
ONEIDA COUNTY
Central New York/Rome
Voluntary Action Center
City Hall on the Mall
Rome 13440

ROCHESTER
Life Line
Health Association of
Rochester and Monroe
County, Inc.
973 East Avenue
Rochester 14607

SCHENECTADY COUNTY
Infoline
432 State Street,
Room 220
Schenectady 12305

SUFFOLK COUNTY
Ask Information and
Referral Service
Suffolk County Department of Social Service
10 Oval Drive
Hauppauge 11787

Suffolk Community
Council, Inc.
1 Edgewood Avenue
Smithtown 11787

WASHINGTON MILLS
Calls for Action
Sponsored by WTLB
   Radio
Kellogg Road
Washington Mills 13479

WATKINS GLEN
Schuyler County Infor-
   mation and Referral
   County Office Building
Watkins Glen 14891

WESTCHESTER COUNTY
Westchester Community
   Service Council, Inc.
237 Mamaroneck Avenue
White Plains 10605

North Carolina

CHARLOTTE
Contact Telephone Coun-
   seling Service
501 North Tryon Street
Charlotte 28202

Information and Referral
   Service
301 South Brevard Street
Charlotte 28202

GREENSBORO
Guilford Information
   and Referral Program

P.O. Box 3388
Greensboro 27402

RALEIGH
Wake County Informa-
   tion and Referral Center
Wake County Public
   Libraries
104 Fayetteville Street
Raleigh 27601

WINSTON-SALEM
First Line
660 West Fifth Street
Winston-Salem 27101

North Dakota

BISMARCK
Information and Referral
   Center
Veterans Memorial Public
   Library
520 Avenue A East
Bismarck 58501

FARGO
Info-Line: Information
   and Referral Service
P.O. Box 732
305 South Eleventh Street
Fargo 58107

Ohio

AKRON
Info Line, Inc.
55 West State Street
Akron 44308

CINCINNATI
Information and Referral
   Center
2400 Reading Road
Cincinnati 45202

CLEVELAND
Community Information
   Service
1005 Huron Road
Cleveland 44115

DAYTON
Information and Referral
   Service: United Way,
   Inc., of the Dayton Area
184 Salem Avenue
Dayton 45406

TOLEDO
Information and Referral
   Center
1 Stanahan Square,
   Room 141
Toledo 43604

Oklahoma

TULSA
Helpline
1430 South Boulder
Tulsa 74119

Oregon

EUGENE
Information and Referral
   Service/Ride Share
   Service
Eugene Switchboard
795 Willamette,
   Room 222
Eugene 97401

PORTLAND
Information and Referral
   Services
Tri-County Community
   Council
718 West Burnside
Portland 97212

SALEM
City of Salem Referral
   Center
1900 Hines Street South-
   east
Salem 97302

Pennsylvania

<u>Allentown</u>
Valley Wide Help
1244 Hamilton Street
Allentown 18102

<u>Harrisburg</u>
Contact-Harrisburg
900 South Arlington
  Avenue
Harrisburg 17109

Tri-County United Way
One United Way
Harrisburg 17110

<u>Lancaster</u>
Lancaster Information
  Center
630 Janet Avenue
Lancaster 17601

<u>Pittsburgh</u>
Helpline Information and
  Volunteer Services
200 Ross Street
Pittsburgh 15219

<u>Reading</u>
Help
Berkshire Towers,
  Suite 236
101 North Fifth Street
Reading 19601

<u>Scranton</u>
FIRST (Free Information
  and Referral System
  Telephone)
200 Adams Avenue
Scranton 18503

<u>Wilkes-Barre</u>
Help Line
73 West Union Street
Wilkes-Barre 18702

Rhode Island

<u>Providence</u>
Council for Community
  Services
Information Service
229 Waterman Street
Providence 02906

South Carolina

<u>Charleston</u>
Trident United Way In-
  formation and Referral
  Service
P.O. Box 2696
Charleston 29403

<u>Columbia</u>
United Way of the
  Midlands
Information and Referral
  Center

P.O. Box 152
Columbia 29202

South Dakota

PIERRE
Pierre Area Referral
  Service
115 South Pierre Street
Pierre 57501

RAPID CITY
Rapid City Volunteer and
  Information Center
517 Seventh Street
Rapid City 57701

SIOUX FALLS
Community Information
  Center
470 Boyce Greeley
  Building
Sioux Falls 57102

Tennessee

CHATTANOOGA
Information and Referral
  Service
Tennessee Department of
  Public Health
Chattanooga 37406

Senior Neighbors, Inc.
Tenth and Newby Streets
Chattanooga 37402

MEMPHIS
Linc Service: Memphis-
  Shelby County Public
  Library and Informa-
  tion Center
1850 Peabody
Memphis 38104

NASHVILLE
CCS Info
250 Venture Circle
Nashville 37228

Texas

DALLAS
Community Council of
  Greater Dallas: Informa-
  tion and Referral Service
1900 Pacific Building,
  Suite 1725
Dallas 75201

FORT WORTH
United Way of Metropoli-
  tan Tarrant County
210 East Ninth Street
Fort Worth 76102

HOUSTON
United Way Information
  and Referral
P.O. Box 13668
Houston 77019

SAN ANTONIO
Help Line
406 West Market
San Antonio 78205

Utah

OGDEN
Weber County Depart-
ment of Human Services:
Information and Referral
Service
2510 Washington
Boulevard, Suite 202
Ogden 84401

PROVO
Utah County Information
and Referral Service
420 North 200 West,
No. 2
Provo 84601

SALT LAKE CITY
Information Center
2900 South Main Street
Salt Lake City 84115

Virginia

ALEXANDRIA
Department of Social
Services: Information
and Referral Service

110 North Royal Street
Alexandria 22314

ARLINGTON
Information and Referral
Department of Human
Services
Arlington County
1800 North Edison Street
Arlington 22207

NEWPORT NEWS
Contact Peninsula, Inc.
211 32nd Street
Newport News 23607

RICHMOND
United Way Information
and Referral Service
2501 Monument Avenue
Richmond 23220

SOUTHEASTERN REGION
Information Center of
Hampton Roads
101 St. Paul's Boulevard
Norfolk 23510

Washington

SEATTLE
Community Information
Line
A Program of Crisis
Clinic, Inc.

1530 Eastlake Avenue
East, Suite 301
Seattle 98102

SPOKANE
Information and Referral
Service for Spokane
County
West 906 Main Avenue
Spokane 99201

TACOMA
Information and Referral
P.O. Box 5007
Tacoma 98405

West Virginia

CHARLESTON
Link Line: Information
and Referral Bureau
Community Council of
Kanawha Valley
P.O. Box 2711
702½ Lee Street
Charleston 25330

HUNTINGTON
Contact
520 Eleventh Street
Huntington 25701

Wisconsin

MADISON
Information and Referral
Providers of Wisconsin,
Inc.
210 Monona Avenue
Madison 53709

United Way of Dane
County
2059 Atwood Avenue
Madison 53704

MILWAUKEE
Hotlines Council of
Southeastern Wiscon-
sin, Inc.
P.O. Box 11565
Milwaukee 53211

Information Service for
the Aging
4420 West Vliet Street
Milwaukee 53208

Wisconsin Information
Service
161 West Wisconsin
Avenue, Room 7075
Milwaukee 53211

Wyoming

CHEYENNE

Volunteer Information
  Center
P.O. Box 404
Cheyenne 82001

Wyoming Information
  and Referral Service, Inc.
1750 Westland Road
Cheyenne 82001

CANADA

Alberta

CALGARY

Advice, Information, and
  Direction Center
229-7 Avenue Southeast
Calgary, Alberta

EDMONTON

Aid Service of Edmonton
203, 10711-107 Avenue
Edmonton T5H 0W6

British Columbia

VANCOUVER

Greater Vancouver Information and Referral Service
105-1956 West Broadway
Vancouver V6J 1Z2

Manitoba

WINNIPEG

United Way of Winnipeg
  Referral Agent Program
315-267 Edmonton Street
Winnipeg R3C 1S2

Nova Scotia

HALIFAX

Help Line
6136 University Avenue
Halifax B3H 4J2

Ontario

HAMILTON

Community Information
  Service
Hamilton-Wentworth
42 James Street North
Suite 609
Hamilton L8R 2K2

OTTAWA

Community Information
  Centre of Ottawa-
  Carleton
377 Rideau Street
Ottawa K1N 5Y6

TORONTO

Community Information
  Centre of Metropolitan
  Toronto

34 King Street East,
  Third Floor
Toronto M5C 1E5

Windsor-Essex Commu-
  nity Information Service
65 Wyandotte Street West
Windsor N9A 5W6

Quebec

MONTREAL
Centre de Réference du
  Grand Montréal/Informa-
  tion and Referral Service
  of Greater Montreal
1800 Dorchester
  Boulevard West
Montreal H3H 2H2

STATE AGENCIES ON AGING

Some families find it helpful to contact the nearest office
for the aging, or area agency on aging, which is funded by
the federal government. You may find this by asking the
telephone information operator, or consulting the telephone directory under the name of your city or county.
States may have different designations for this office, so I
have provided this list of state agencies to help you find
the one nearest you.

Alabama
Commission on Aging
740 Madison Avenue
Montgomery 36104
(205) 832-6640

Alaska
Office on Aging
Dept. of Health and
  Social Services

Pouch H
Juneau 99811
(907) 586-6153

Arizona
Bureau on Aging
Dept. of Economic
  Security
543 East McDowell,
  Room 217

Phoenix 85004
(602) 271-4446

Arkansas
Office on Aging and
Adult Services
Dept. of Human Services
7107 West 12th
P.O. Box 2179
Little Rock 72203
(501) 371-2441

California
Dept. of Aging
Health and Welfare
Agency
918 J Street
Sacramento 95814
(916) 322-3887

Colorado
Division of Services for
the Aging
Dept. of Social Services
1575 Sherman St.
Denver 80203
(303) 892-2651

Connecticut
Dept. on Aging
90 Washington St.,
Rm. 312
Hartford 06115
(203) 566-7725

Delaware
Division of Aging
Dept. of Health and
Social Services
2413 Lancaster Avenue
Wilmington 19805
(302) 571-3481

District of Columbia
Office of Aging
Office of the Mayor,
Suite 1106
1012 14th St., N.W.
Washington, D.C. 20005
(202) 724-5623

Florida
Program Office of Aging
and Adult Services
Dept. of Health and
Rehabilitation Services
1323 Winewood Blvd.
Tallahassee 32301
(904) 488-2650

Georgia
Office of Aging
Dept. of Human
Resources
610 Ponce de Leon Ave.,
N.E.
Atlanta 30308
(404) 894-5333

Hawaii
Executive Office on
  Aging
1149 Bethel St., Rm. 311
Honolulu 96813
(808) 548-2593

Idaho
Idaho Office on Aging
Statehouse
Boise 83720
(208) 384-3833

Illinois
Dept. on Aging
2401 West Jefferson
Springfield 62706
(217) 782-5773

Indiana
Commission on Aging
  and Aged
Graphic Arts Bldg.
215 North Senate Avenue
Indianapolis 46202
(317) 633-5948

Iowa
Commission on Aging
Jewett Bldg.
415 West 10th St.
Des Moines 50319
(515) 281-5187

Kansas
Department of Aging
Biddle Building
2700 W. 6th St.
Topeka 66606
(913) 296-4986

Kentucky
Center for Aging and
  Community Development
Dept. for Human
  Resources
403 Wapping St.
Frankfort 40601
(502) 564-6930

Louisiana
Bureau of Aging Services
Division of Human
  Resources
Health and Human
  Resources Administration
P.O. Box 44282
  Capitol Station
Baton Rouge 70804
(504) 389-2171

Maine
Bureau of Maine's Elderly
Community Services Unit
Dept. of Human Services
State House
Augusta 04333
(207) 289-2561

Maryland
Office on Aging
State Office Bldg.
301 West Preston St.
Baltimore 21201
(301) 383-5064

Massachusetts
Dept. of Elder Affairs
110 Tremont St.
Boston 02108
(617) 727-7750

Michigan
Office of Services to the
   Aging
300 East Michigan
P.O. Box 30026
Lansing 48909
(517) 373-8230

Minnesota
Governor's Citizens
   Council on Aging,
   Suite 204
Metro Square Bldg.
7th and Robert Sts.
St. Paul 55101
(612) 296-2544

Mississippi
Council on Aging
P.O. Box 5136
Fondren Station

510 George St.
Jackson 39216
(601) 354-6590

Missouri
Office of Aging
Division of Special
   Services
Dept. of Social Services
Broadway State Office
   Bldg.
P.O. Box 570
Jefferson City 65101
(314) 751-2075

Montana
Aging Services Bureau
Dept. of Social and
   Rehabilitation Services
P.O. Box 1723
Helena 59601
(406) 449-3124

Nebraska
Commission on Aging
State House Station 94784
P.O. Box 95044
Lincoln 68509
(402) 471-2307

Nevada
Division of Aging
   Services

Dept. of Human
  Resources
Kinkead Bldg., Rm. 600
505 East King Street
Carson City 89710
(702) 885-4210

New Hampshire
Council on Aging
P.O. Box 786
14 Depot St.
Concord 03301
(603) 271-2751

New Jersey
Division on Aging
Dept. of Community
  Affairs
P.O. Box 2768
363 West State St.
Trenton 08625
(609) 292-4833

New Mexico
Commission on Aging
408 Galisteo–Villagra
  Bldg.
Santa Fe 87503
(505) 827-5258

New York
Office for the Aging
Agency Bldg. 2
Empire State Plaza

Albany 12223
(518) 474-5731

**New York City Field
Office**
2 World Trade Center,
  Room 5036
New York City 10047
(212) 488-6405

North Carolina
North Carolina Div. for
  Aging
Dept. of Health
  Resources
213 Hillsborough St.
Raleigh 27603
(919) 733-3983

North Dakota
Aging Services
Social Services Board of
  N.D.
State Capitol Bldg.
Bismarck 58505
(701) 224-2577

Ohio
Commission on Aging
50 West Broad St.
Columbus 43216
(614) 466-5500

Oklahoma
Special Unit on Aging
Department of Institutions, Social and Rehabilitation Services
P.O. Box 25352
Oklahoma City 73125
(405) 521-2281

Oregon
Program on Aging
Human Resources Dept.
772 Commercial St., S.E.
Salem 97310
(503) 378-4728

Pennsylvania
Office for the Aging
Dept. of Public Welfare
Health and Welfare
   Bldg., Rm. 540
P.O. Box 2675
7th and Forster Sts.
Harrisburg 17120
(717) 787-5350

Rhode Island
Division on Aging
Department of
   Community Affairs
150 Washington Ct.
Providence 02903
(401) 277-2858

Samoa
Territorial Administration
   on Aging
Government of American
   Samoa
Pago Pago,
American Samoa 96799

South Carolina
Commission on Aging
915 Main St.
Columbia 29201
(803) 758-2576

South Dakota
Office on Aging
Dept. of Social Services
State Office Bldg.
Illinois Street
Pierre 57501
(605) 224-3656

Tennessee
Commission on Aging
S&P Bldg., Room 201
306 Gay Street
Nashville 37201
(615) 741-2056

Texas
Governor's Committee
   on Aging
Exec. Office Bldg., Fls. 4&5

411 W. 13th St.
Austin 78703
(512) 475-2717

Utah
Division of Aging
Dept. of Social Services
150 West North Temple
Salt Lake City 84102
(801) 533-6422

Vermont
Office on Aging
Agency of Human
  Services
81 River St. (Heritage 1)
Montpelier 05602
(802) 828-3471

Washington
Office on Aging
Dept. of Social and
  Health Services
P.O. Box 1788—M.S.
  45-2
Olympia 98504
(206) 753-2502

West Virginia
Commission on Aging
State Capitol
Charleston 25305
(304) 348-3317

Wisconsin
Division on Aging
Dept. of Health and
  Social Services
1 West Wilson St.,
  Rm. 686
Madison 53703
(608) 266-2536

Wyoming
Aging Services
Dept. of Health and
  Social Services
Division of Public Assis-
  tance and Social Services
New State Office Bldg. West,
  Rm. 288
Cheyenne 82002

COUNSELING SERVICES

There are some private social workers and psychologists
who are specialists in helping older people and their fami-

lies, usually called gerontological social workers or geriatric counselors. However, this specialty is so new that there is not as yet any list available of qualified practitioners.

Counseling on social, emotional, and practical problems may be obtained through many sources. I suggest first locating a family service agency near you. Check in the Yellow Pages of the telephone directory under Social Service Agencies or Organizations.

The following list is suggestive of how you may start your investigation:

> Catholic Services to the Elderly
> Christian Community Service Organization
> Jewish Family and Children's Services
> United Family and Children's Services

Counseling is also available through:

> hospital social work departments
> mental health clinics
> churches and synagogues
> senior citizen centers
> senior housing
> long-term care facilities

Many other health and welfare organizations offer counseling as part of their services.

HOMEMAKERS/AIDES OR ATTENDANTS

Finding and retaining reliable help to care for the mentally impaired aged at home is a constant problem for some families. Once again, the first step should be a call to the local ADRDA chapter. Families can pass on leads to others as to which help is reliable.

The other sources for specialized staff who are trained to work with the mentally impaired aged are homemaker/home health agencies, visiting nurse associations, and public health nursing associations.

These services can be very expensive, and are a problem for many families. For those eligible for Medicaid, some home health services may be available on a limited basis, if it is determined that otherwise the older person would have to be institutionalized. Check with your local Medicaid office to see if your relative is eligible for any programs that are considered "alternatives to institutionalization."

HELP WITH FINANCES OR HEALTH CARE EXPENSES

Your local Social Security office has counselors who can provide you with information on Medicare benefits (help with certain medical expenses) and supplemental security income (SSI) for the indigent elderly and handicapped. Be sure to have your relative's social security number available when you call, or visit the office in person.

For information on Medicaid (health-care benefits for the indigent elderly and handicapped) you will have to contact your local welfare office. The name for this office varies from state to state, and even from city to county. They all come under the United States Department of Health and Human Services (DHHS), but they may be called Department of Health and Human Resources, Human Resources Department, Department of Public Social Services, etc. Be prepared to document information about your relative's finances with bank statements, copies of income checks, proof of age and residency, and so forth.

LEGAL SERVICES

Some concerns of families of the mentally impaired aged present complex legal and ethical challenges that may be beyond the experience of many attorneys. If you have such problems, try to locate an attorney who is experienced in protective custody, commitments, conservatorship, and other such issues. A call to the Bar Association, or to the office for the aging, should provide a referral to several reliable attorneys who can help.

If you and your relative are without adequate funds to pay legal fees, check with your local office for the aging to ascertain whether they have an office for legal services to the elderly, or if there is a division of Legal Aid that can help with problems of the elderly.

Your local office of the Department of Health and Human Services may have a Protective Services Division. They are usually knowledgeable and helpful about many of the legal issues concerning the mentally impaired.

APPENDIX 4

Selected Drugs for Common Problems in Old Age That Can Cause Symptoms of Mental Impairment

D rugs may be known by registered brand names, or by their generic chemical names. The following table lists some of the prescription drugs frequently taken by older people for common health problems, and that can cause symptoms of mental impairment as unintended side effects. It is important to know that some nonprescription drugs, such as antihistamine preparations for colds, can also cause confusion and even hallucinations as side effects in some elderly persons. Also, alcohol, which is much more commonly used by older people than is usually recognized, can cause mental impairment when taken alone or in conjunction with other drugs.

The principle to keep in mind is to raise questions with the physician about any drug taken by your relative who may have recently developed symptoms of mental impairment or whose mental function has noticeably changed.

Diagnosis	Medication	Possible Side Effects
high blood pressure and heart conditions	Aldomet Aldoril Diuril Diupres Hydrodiuril Hydropres Hygroton Inderal Lasix Regroton Reserpine Serpasil	confusion, memory loss, depression
heart conditions	Digitalis Digoxin Lanoxin Inderal	confusion, depression, disorientation, nervousness, hallucinations
depression	Aventyl Elavil Parnate Pertofrane Lithium Ritalin Sinequan Tofranil	memory loss, confusion, anxiety, agitation, delirium, disorientation, paranoia, hallucinations
nervousness, anxiety	Ativan Librium Serax Tranxene Valium	confusion, memory loss, depression

Diagnosis	Medication	Possible Side Effects
sleeping problems	chloral hydrate Dalmane Phenobarbital Quaalude Seconal	confusion, depression
Parkinson's disease	Artane Levodopa (L-Dopa) Sinemet Symmetral	forgetfulness, confusion, hallucinations, paranoia
arthritis	Aristocort Butazolidin cortisone Hydrocortone Indocin Prednisone	depression, psychosis, paranoia
diabetes	insulin Orinase	acute mental changes
ulcers	Tagamet if taken with Inderal Tagamet if taken with Valium Tagamet if taken with Aminophyllin (for asthma)	short-term memory loss, disorientation, anxiety, depression
pain	Tylenol with Codeine Phenacetin	Agitation, hallucinations, depression

APPENDIX 5

Nursing Home Staff

Total number of these personnel is related to number of beds in the facility.

Administrator: Responsible for overall management of facility, to health department and board (if voluntary, nonprofit) or owner (if proprietary, private).

Physician(s): Responsible for medical care of residents/patients.

Director of nursing: Responsible for overall nursing care of residents/patients.

Nursing supervisor: Gives direct patient care and supervises care given by other RNs (registered nurses), LPNs (licensed practical nurses) and aides/orderlies (attendants).

Charge nurse: Responsible for a specific area—nursing floor, section, etc. May or may not be the nursing supervisor.

Registered nurse: More professional education, more autonomy in practice than licensed practical nurse; both levels of professionals carry out nursing plans, administer medications, observe and monitor patients.

Aides: Provide direct care to patients/residents: bathing, dressing, grooming, toileting, making beds, feeding, etc.

Orderlies/attendants: Provide same services as aides, usually for male residents/patients.

Admissions personnel: Provide information and applications prior to admission, and arrange for contract upon admission to institution. In some institutions this function is part of the social work department, and involves intake interview to determine appropriateness of application.

Social worker: Professional responsible for assessing and planning for the social and psychological needs of residents/patients.

Social work assistant (sometimes called social work designee): Works under the supervision of the social worker to provide for the psychosocial needs of residents/patients.

Recreation worker: Responsible for a planned therapeutic activity program.

Dietician: Plans and supervises meals and special diets.

Kitchen staff: prepares meals.

Housekeeping staff: Cleans patients'/residents' rooms and public areas.

Business office: Handles billing, personal allowances, etc.

Larger nursing homes may also have:

Psychiatrist(s): to diagnose and treat mental health needs.

Occupational therapist: to assess resident/patient function in activities of daily living, and plan and carry out treatment programs.

Physical therapist: to implement physical therapy under physician's orders, such as exercise programs, heat and massage treatment, etc.

Speech therapist: to assess and treat for speech impairments.

Pharmacist: to dispense medications and medical supplies, and in some institutions to supervise medication management.

Clergy: to meet spiritual needs of residents and their families.

Volunteer director: to recruit and supervise volunteers who provide a wide range of services including friendly visiting, reading and writing letters for residents, organizing individualized activities, shopping, etc.

GLOSSARY OF SELECTED TERMS

Alzheimer's disease A degenerative brain disorder, involving disruption of neurotransmitter activity, the cause of which is unknown. When it occurs before age 65 it is called presenile dementia; after 65 it is called senile dementia—Alzheimer's type. It is characterized by severe memory impairment, confusion, disorientation, behavioral changes, and progressive disintegration of the personality.

Ambulatory Able to walk, with or without assistance. Often a criterion used in nursing assessments.

Aphasia Loss of the ability to use words due to brain damage. This can take the form of inability to express thoughts, or to understand what is being said.

Dehydration A condition in which the body is abnormally depleted of fluids, sometimes resulting in mental impairment.

Delusion An abnormal mental state in which false ideas are believed to be true in spite of the facts.

Dementia Deterioration of the brain resulting in impaired intellect, memory, and willpower; behavior may be confused and irrational.

Diuretics Medications that increase urination with the purpose of decreasing excess fluids in the body. Often prescribed for high blood pressure and heart conditions. Sometimes lead to an imbalance of essential minerals, such as potassium, which, if not replaced, can cause symptoms of mental impairment and other problems.

Electroshock treatment When drug therapy has not helped to alleviate the symptoms of severe depressive illness, the use of electrically induced seizures can be very effective. The patient is tranquilized and premedicated to prevent cardiac complications; a fast-acting anesthetic is used, and treatment lasts less than a minute. After the seizure is over, oxygen is administered and the patient quickly regains consciousness, with no recollection of the treatment. Some memory impairment results at the same time that the depressive symptoms lift, but the memory loss usually improves a few weeks after the electroshock treatment.

Geriatrics The branch of medicine that provides health care to the aged.

Gerontology The interdisciplinary study of aging in society, encompassing social, economic, physiological, and psychological changes over the life span.

Incompetency Legal status of a person who is unable to manage his affairs because of a mental or physical impairment, as determined by court. The definition varies according to each state's statutes as interpreted by the courts. Court declaration of incompetency will result in the appointment of a guardian who will take care of managing the incompetent's property, with accountability to the court.

Incontinence Inability to contain or control urination or defecation (bowel movement). Usually differentiated as urinary incontinence or fecal incontinence.

Medicaid A medical benefits program for the elderly and disabled who are indigent. This federal program is administered by the states, with varying reimbursement rates, resulting in unequal eligibility requirements and benefits from one state to another. Specific information on coverage and eligibility can be obtained from the local office of the Department of Health and Human Services.

Medicare A federal health insurance program designed to provide hospital care (Part A) and supplemental medical benefits (Part B) for persons age 65 and over, regardless of income level. Beneficiaries must pay a deductible fee and percentage of costs (co-insurance), as well as monthly premiums if they want Part B coverage. These costs have increased drastically since Medicare started in 1965, and many older people carry supplementary insurance, such as Blue Cross and Blue Shield, to help meet these costs. Information on current benefits and costs can be obtained from the Social Security Administration.

Mental impairment A state of mental dysfunction in which there are problems with memory, moods, understanding, and behavior, which may be the result of a variety of conditions; some may be chronic and irreversible, others acute, treatable, and reversible.

Multi-infarct dementia Mental deterioration due to blood vessel disease in the brain. Symptoms are caused by the progressive damage of strokes, or the cutting off of oxygen to the brain by a blood clot, a spasm, or the rupture of an artery. The damage to tissue deprived of oxygen is called an infarct. This damage can also accumulate as a result of transient ischemic attacks (TIAs), sometimes called "little strokes." Ischemia is the cutting off of oxygen. TIAs are often barely noticeable, and may take the form of temporary paralysis or numbness, sudden but temporary memory gaps, transitory weakness, slurred speech, etc.

Neurofibrillary tangles An abnormal accumulation of damaged fibers found in the nerve cells of the brain in Alzheimer's disease. Its cause is unknown, as well as its specific effect. It is known only that the greater the accumulation of tangles and plaques (which are the result of degeneration of nerve endings), the more severe the symptoms of dementia.

Neurotransmitters Chemicals secreted by specific nerve cells to communicate or pass messages to other nerve cells. Neurotransmitters such as acetylcholine are manufactured in the neurons that secrete them, and enzymes such as choline acetyltransferase are needed to catalyze these chemical reactions. In Alzheimer's disease there is a marked decrease in acetylcholine in the part of the brain that involves memory.

Organic brain syndrome Mental, emotional, and behavioral symptoms caused by physiological changes in the brain. This term is used synonymously with dementia.

Paranoia A condition of disordered thinking in which a person suffers delusions of persecution, morbid jealousy, and grandeur, among other symptoms. The delusions are typically persistent and systematized, and usually can be understood as compensating for mental and sensory changes that create some anxiety. If one responds to the feelings of anxiety, this usually is helpful to an elderly person, and the paranoid state may be of shorter duration than in younger persons. Chronic paranoid states are usually responsive to major tranquilizers.

Pseudodementia A condition that mimics dementia in that the same symptoms of mental, emotional, and behavioral changes may be present. However, it is caused by a condition that is reversible if treated. Most pseudodementia is caused by depression or drug toxicity. Other frequent causes are chemical imbalances due to dehydration, malnutrition, anemia, and thyroid dysfunction. Chronic heart and lung conditions can deprive the brain of oxygen, causing pseudodementia.

Reversible brain syndrome Another term for pseudodementia.

Senility A commonly used term to describe the abnormal mental and physical deterioration of old age. It often reflects a negative and hopeless attitude about aging that ignores the fact that abnormal changes are caused by specific medical conditions, and are not typical of the normal aging process.

Supplemental Security Income (SSI) A federal cash payment program for the elderly or disabled whose income falls below an established eligibility level. It is handled by the Social Security Administration and financed through general taxes. Many states add funds to the base amount paid by the federal government. Information and applications are available through the local office of the Social Security Administration.

RECOMMENDED READING AND SELECTED BIBLIOGRAPHY

Because the problems we have covered are so complex, no book can presume to supply all of the answers, or even all of the directions toward answers. (Sometimes all you can hope to learn is how not to make a bad situation worse!) The following books are recommended for you to read as a course of study. Each will provide you with a body of information that will help you obtain a broader view of the issues affecting you and your impaired older relative.

RECOMMENDED READING

Benowicz, Robert. *Vitamins and You* (New York: Berkley Books, 1981). This is a very useful guide to vitamins and minerals, particularly important in meeting nutritional needs of the elderly.

Butler, Robert. *Why Survive? Being Old in America* (New York: Harper & Row, 1975). Pulitzer Prize–winning overview of the impact of aging in contemporary America.

Cammer, Leonard, M.D. *Up From Depression* (New York: Simon and Schuster, 1969). A psychiatrist's overview of depressive illness and treatment, with special emphasis on the family's role.

Freese, Arthur S. *Stroke! The New Hope and the New Help* (New York: Random House, 1980). A very thorough examination of the nature of stroke and its treatment.

Galton, Lawrence, *The Truth About Senility and How to Avoid It* (New York: Thomas Y. Crowell, 1979). Although the title is misleading, this fact-filled book about other conditions that cause symptoms imitating senility can be very useful to anyone who questions the diagnosis of his mentally impaired older relative.

Graedon, Joe. *The People's Pharmacy 2.* (New York: Avon Books, 1980). An invaluable aid in understanding medications and their possible effects and side effects, a very important skill when it is necessary to be knowledgeable about your relative's drug regimen.

Mace, Nancy, and Peter Rabins, M.D. *The 36-Hour Day: A Family Guide to Caring for Persons with Alzheimer's Disease, Related Dementing Illnesses and Memory Loss in Later Life.* (Baltimore: John Hopkins University Press, 1981). A must-read book for those families caring for the mentally impaired person at home. Filled with practical advice on problems of home care, it also provides insights into the emotional stresses involved and offers constructive suggestions for dealing with them.

Mindell, Earl. *Earl Mindell's Vitamin Bible* (New York: Warner Books, 1979). Another helpful guide to nutritional supplements.

Otten, Jane, and Florence Shelly. *When Your Parents Grow Old*. (New York: Signet, 1976). An informative guide to resources for problems confronting families of the aging, particularly the normally alert, mentally intact. The excellent practical advice in such areas as money matters, health care, and communication with doctors is also applicable to families of the mentally impaired aged.

Reisberg, Barry, M.D. *Brain Failure: An Introduction to Current Concepts of Senility* (New York: Free Press, 1981). A text designed to provide professionals in the health field with an updated overview of senile dementia. Despite technical terminology and medical language, this book is easy to read, and it can provide a comprehensive understanding of the physiology of brain failure that causes mental and physical impairment in old age.

Silverstone, Barbara, and Helen Hyman. *You and Your Aging Parent: The Modern Family's Guide to Emotional, Physical, and Financial Problems*. (New York: Pantheon, 1976). The most readable, understanding presentation of the emotional impact on middle-aged children as their parents become dependent. Its focus is on relationships with parents who are alert, but principles can be applied to a broad range of family situations.

Williams, Roger. *Nutrition Against Disease* (New York: Bantam, 1981). A classic to help you understand the relationship of nutrition to health and illness.

SELECTED BIBLIOGRAPHY

Birren, James E., and Bruce Sloane, eds. *Handbook of Mental Health and Aging.* Englewood Cliffs, New Jersey: Prentice-Hall, 1980.

Blumenthal, Monica. "Depressive Illness in Old Age: Getting Behind the Mask." *Geriatrics*, April 1980.

Brody, Elaine. "Aging and Family Personality: A Developmental View." *Family Process* 13, no. 1 (March 1971).

————. "The Aging Family," *Gerontologist* 6, no. 4 (1966).

Busse, Ewald, and Eric Pfeiffer. *Behavior and Adaptation in Later Life.* Boston: Little, Brown, 1969.

————. *Mental Illness in Later Life.* Washington: American Psychiatric Association, 1973.

Butler, Robert, and Myrna Lewis. *Aging and Mental Health: Positive Psychosocial Approaches.* St. Louis: C. V. Mosby Co., 1973.

Caplan, Gerald, and Marie Killilea, *Support Systems and Mutual Help.* New York: Grune and Stratton, 1976.

Cowdry, E. V., ed. *The Care of the Geriatric Patient.* St. Louis: C. V. Mosby Co., 1968.

Davis, Richard, and William Smith, eds. *Drugs and the Elderly.* Los Angeles: Ethel Percy Andrus Gerontology Center, University of Southern California, 1973.

Dobrof, Rose, and Eugene Litwak. *Maintenance of Family Ties of Long-Term Care Patients: Theory and Guide to Practice.* Rockville, Maryland: National Institute of Mental Health, 1977.

Eisdorfer, Carl. "Observations on the Psychopharmacology of the Aged," *Journal of the American Geriatrics Society* 23, no. 2 (February 1975).

Eisdorfer, Carl, and Robert Friedl, eds. *Cognitive and Emotional Disturbances in the Elderly.* Chicago: Year Book Medical Publishing Co., 1977.

Katzman, Robert, et al., eds. *Alzheimer's Disease: Senile Dementia and Related Disorders.* New York: Raven Press, 1978.

Kline, Nathan, ed. *Factors in Depression.* New York: Raven Press, 1974.

Kral, V. A. "Senile Dementia and Normal Aging." *Canadian Psychiatric Association Journal* 17, no. 11 (1972).

Lindemann, Eric. "Symptomatology and Management of Acute Grief." *American Journal of Psychiatry* 101 (1944).

MacMillan, Duncan. "Features of Senile Breakdown." *Geriatrics* 24 (March 1969).

Managing the Disturbed Elderly Patient in Family Practice. Fort Washington, Pennsylvania: McNeil Laboratories, 1977.

Reisberg, Barry. *Brain Failure: An Introduction to Current Concepts of Senility.* New York: Free Press, 1981.

Schoenberg, Bernard, et al., eds. *Psychosocial Aspects of Terminal Care.* New York: Columbia University Press, 1972.

Schorr, Alvin. *Filial Responsibility in the American Family.* Washington, D.C.: U.S. Government Printing Office, 1960.

Shanas, Ethel, and Gordon Streib, eds. *Social Structure and the Family: Generational Relations.* Englewood Cliffs, New Jersey: Prentice-Hall, 1965.

Whitehead, J. M. *Psychiatric Disorders in Old Age: A Handbook for the Clinical Team.* New York: Springer, 1974.

INDEX

comfortable quarters in, 213–14

decision to place elder in, *see* Institutionalization

family councils for, 210, 243–45

family's relation to and interaction with, 210, 215–16, 217–19, 227–28

health of residents in, 235–36, 237–39

interview of applicants by, 199–200

level of care in, 196–98

locating suitable one, 194–203

location of, 201–2

neglect in, 228–32

number of, in U.S., 206

overt sexual behavior in, 164

private vs. public, 208

problems and complaints in, 220–28

prolonging life in, 237–39

rating scales of, 196–97

regulation of, 208

restraint of residents in, 230

roommates in, 219–20

segregation of mentally impaired in, 198–99

staff of, *see* Nursing-home staff

support groups formed at, 242–43

as a system, 208–12

transfers among, 202

treatment plan in, 217–20

visiting, 232–34

Nursing-home staff, 208–11, 215–17

aides and attendants, 211, 216

anger at and jealousy of, 235

and anxiety of elderly moving to facility, 203, 207, 213

appreciation of, 232

criticism of, 209–210, 216, 227–28

personnel of (listing), 299–301

and sexual behavior of residents, 164–65

volunteer, 211, 227

Nutrition

and depression, 61

needs, of elderly living alone, 260

see also Malnutrition

Nutrition programs, 66

Observation of older person

for diagnosis of incontinence, 157

for diagnosis of mental impairment, 72–73, 90, 91

on medications, 61–62, 69–70, 168

of moods, 37

of smoking, for safety, 129

Obstinacy, 31–32, 160; *see also* Cooperation of elder, lack of

Organic brain syndrome (OBS), 12–13, 14, 305–6

Organic mental syndrome (OMS), 12

Orientation, failures of, *see* Disorientation

Paranoia, 34–35, 138–54, 306

Parkinson's disease, 55–56, 298

Perceptual changes, 42–43

Perseveration, 24, 39

Physical examination

for diagnosis, 96

for new nursing-home resident, 217

for nursing-home admittance, 199, 200